Beyond Recog
A Critique of Contemporary S

Neal Harris

Contents

Introduction

On the Importance and Relevance of Social Pathology Scholarship

On the origins and import of this research

Why Social Pathology?

Long before I encountered the concept of social pathology I had been intuitively fascinated by 'deeper', more 'foundational' social critiques. In my teenage years, as a socialist from a working-class family, society simply seemed 'crazy' or 'illogical' to me. I would read about the grotesque inequalities of wealth, the self-indulgent fancies of billionaires, man-made global warming, the continued presence of racial and gender inequalities, neo-colonial wars, even the persistence of the House of Lords ... to my unschooled mind, the best word to describe this was 'bonkers'. So, as a precocious (at times insufferable) college student, I would puzzle over Rousseau and Nietzsche, not always understanding it, but feeling there was 'something' there which was 'weightier' than the prescribed liberal readings of my textbooks. During my undergraduate degree I became fascinated by Hegel and Adorno for similar reasons, and with comparable semi-comprehension. It was only during my Master's, that these thoughts developed any clear form, and I slowly became aware that there was a rich theoretical literature on the explicit commonality across these authors: that of 'social pathology'.

This realisation largely came through reading Axel Honneth, who, at time of writing, is director of the *Institute for Social Research*, the symbolic home of the so-called 'Frankfurt School' of Critical Theory. Indeed, from one perspective, the reader might engage with this thesis as borne out of a 'love-hate' relationship with Honneth's output, and his increasing divergence from earlier generations of Critical Theory (Honneth, 2000, 2004a, 2007a, 2010, 2014a). Two of Honneth's lesser known texts were central to drawing me into the literature on social pathology diagnosis. Honneth's (2004a) 'A social pathology of reason: on the Intellectual legacy of Critical Theory' and his (2014a) 'The diseases of society: Approaching a nearly impossible concept' seemed to articulate with superb clarity the importance of diagnosing social pathologies and expertly illuminated what this tradition has represented. Yet, simultaneously, Honneth's own substantive scholarship seemed increasingly restrictive, even reactionary. The more I studied them, Honneth's *The Struggle for Recognition* (1995) and particularly his *Freedom's Right* (2014) seemed entirely incommensurate with the theoretical insights and political urgency of earlier generations of Critical Theory. Honneth thus annoyed me, he seemed to 'get it', but not to 'do it' when it came to diagnosing social pathologies.

Mid-way through the first term of my doctoral research, Michael J. Thompson's *The Domestication of Critical Theory* was published. I found myself in broad agreement with his argument: contemporary Critical Theory was a far cry from the political and philosophical radicalism of earlier generations. Thompson's (2016) powerful argument, that Critical Theory has suffered a process of 'domestication', fitted perfectly with my own, protean thoughts on social pathology scholarship. Having read Thompson's text repeatedly the central idea of this thesis became settled, to show how contemporary scholarship on social pathology has led to a domestication of this crucial area of Critical Theoretical research.

From these foundations the ideas which developed into this project began to crystallise: diagnosing the central irrationalities of the social conjecture, the 'social pathologies', remains a crucial, if not t*he* crucial task for Critical Theory, yet contemporary Critical Theorists were failing to do it adequately. Largely, this seemed to be due to the turn to a needlessly restrictive, and philosophically questionable, recognition-derived framework for conducting social theory and social research; an approach furthered largely by Honneth's Critical Theory.

Yet, while demonstrating the limitations and the domesticated nature of contemporary pathology diagnosis was an important goal, like Thompson, I was keen to go further. I wanted to point towards possibilities for renewal and to draw out the occluded potential for social theory and social research residing in the myriad framings of social pathology that have been lost in the recognition turn. My project was thus to have two objectives: to demonstrate the limitations of the dominant recognition-derived approaches to social pathology scholarship, and, perhaps more importantly, to articulate the potency of the multiple framings of social pathology once central to Critical Theoretical scholarship, which have been needlessly jettisoned in the recognition turn. This latter task helps to point towards resources that could be united as part of a broader, non-recognition-restrictive approach to conducting foundational, social pathology diagnosing critique.

One important clarification is required from the start of this project: this is not a trans-historical critique of recognition and its role in social theory and social philosophy. Rather, while I agree entirely with Thompson's critique of the neo-Idealism present within the dominant form of recognition scholarship today, this is not to suggest that all recognition-derived social theory is impotent. Instead, it is the contemporary Honnethian form of recognition theory, which is neo-Idealist and restrictive, and thus damaging to theoretical inquiry. This project has no quarrel with the broader recognition tradition in social theory and social philosophy, indeed the left-Hegelian roots of the Critical Theory project are explicitly triumphed and are pointed to as one amongst several means for potential rejuvenation. As I draw out in the penultimate chapter of this thesis, a drastically reformulated recognition approach could perhaps feature as part of a broader, 'polycentric', pathology diagnosing endeavour (Fraser and Honneth, 2001). Yet, in keeping with McNay (2008), Fraser (Fraser and Honneth, 2001) and Thompson (2016, 2017, 2019), as I draw out throughout this thesis, for recognition theory to play any such a role in Critical Theoretical scholarship, it must cede claims to a monopoly on interpretative capacity and must drop all pretensions to the ontological primacy of the recognition dyad. A reformulated, nuanced recognition approach could indeed play a useful subordinate role in a more radical and rejuvenated Critical Theory, but substantial changes are required.

Thus, the answer to 'Why study social pathology?' is two-fold: first, the diagnosis of social pathologies offers the resources to conduct a potent critique of the social world, which, as I shall establish, enables the theorist to transcend the limited liberal framings of 'justice' and 'legitimacy' (Neuhouser, 2012). Equally, and as will be demonstrated in subsequent chapters, the potency of this tradition is being 'domesticated' (Thompson, 2016). I thus felt drawn to conducting research on this topic, as I wanted to make an intervention to expose how this important area of Critical Theory was being debased, and to reaffirm the utility and critical insight of a potent, unrestricted, pathology diagnosing engagement with the social world.

The Frankfurt School of Critical Theory

The *Institut für Sozialforschung* [Institute for Social Research], home to the 'Frankfurt School', was founded in 1923 as an autonomous research institution affiliated with the University of Frankfurt am Main.[1] Originally uniting mainly orthodox Marxist economists, the institute developed an idiosyncratic interdisciplinary critique, uniting aspects from German Idealism, anti-positivist sociology and psychoanalysis (Jay, 1996). Horkheimer's programmatic essay 'Traditional and Critical Theory' (1937) is perhaps the clearest 'manifesto' for the research project, explicitly articulating the methodological and political commitments of the institute. It is commonplace for academics to talk of 'generations' of Critical Theory, with a first generation of Max Horkheimer, Herbert Marcuse, Theodor W. Adorno, Walter Benjamin, Erich Fromm *inter alia*, a second generation around Jürgen Habermas, a third generation of Axel Honneth and Claus Offe *inter alia*, and today one may even hear of a fourth generation orbiting Rainer Forst.

---

[1] For a detailed and accessible group biography of the Frankfurt School theorists, see Stuart Jeffries' *Grand Hotel Abyss* (2017). For a more rigorous academic history, see Martin Jay's *The Dialectical Imagination* (1973) or David Held's *Introduction to Critical Theory: Horkheimer to Habermas* (2013). For a brief introduction, see Stephen Bronner's (2011) *Critical Theory: A Very Short Introduction*.

As Honneth (2000, 2004a, 2007b, 2007c) has argued, across these generations Critical Theory has long been concerned with the diagnosis of social pathologies. This in part comes from the 'deeper' more 'foundational' nature of its critique (Neuhouser, 2011) which focuses not solely on justice, legitimacy and democracy, but on social rationality and the aims to which society functions (Horkheimer, 1937; Honneth, 2000, 2007b; How, 2003). Drawing on its left-Hegelian heritage, Critical Theory engages with the contradictions latent within the manifest forms of social reason (Marcuse, 1969). It is worth stressing that for first-generation Critical Theorists 'reason' is metaphysical, existing both in the forms of social organisation and in the cognitive capacities of the social subject (Marcuse, 1969).

Borne out of these left-Hegelian roots, Critical Theory evinces a unique fusion of theory and praxis. Through their social critique, Critical Theorists seek to overcome the contradictions present within the social order, both cognitive (through ideology critique) and social-structural (through identifying the sites of domination and extraction in the objective social world) (Strydom, 2011). For Critical Theorists, the diagnosis of social pathologies marks a distinct knowledge interest but also an explicit investment in social praxis. Through diagnosing social pathologies, Critical Theory is how consciousness 'fights back' (Jeffries, 2017).

The explicitly political, forward-looking nature of Critical Theory is further evinced through its unique methodological commitment to immanent-transcendence (Delanty, 2011; Strydom, 2011). As I shall draw out in Chapter Five, Critical Theorists seek to identify in the paradoxes of the present the latent higher forms of reason which are already existing, dormant within the social conjecture. The focus on immanent-transcendence enables Critical Theorists to conduct normatively undergirded critique of the objective social order, pointing to the potential of a more rational future society, while focusing their analysis firmly on the contradictions of the immanent present. Honneth has argued that such an approach is best framed as normative, disclosing and diagnostic (Honneth, 2000). Delanty argues that through immanent transcendence,

> Critical Theory thus gave expression to a moral vision of the future possibilities of society as deriving from a process of social transformation driven forward by its internal dynamics (Delanty, 2011: 72).

As Guess (1981) writes, through immanent-transcendence, with its focus on internal contradictions, Critical Theory provides the methodology for its own self-criticism and thus (theoretically) inculcates a predilection for critical reflexivity. Both with a focus on the Critical Theorist herself, and within society more broadly, the methodology of immanent-transcendence retains its clear left-Hegelian inflection and seeks both 'the transformation of the individual's psyche' (ideology-critique) and 'institutional change' (Delanty, 2011: 72).

In addition to its explicitly forward-looking orientation, Critical Theory is distinguished by a hyper-awareness of its positionality: within ideology, within a capitalist, irrational system. As Horkheimer drew out in his signal essay, 'Traditional and Critical Theory', the project can further be understood as 'critical', as unlike the 'savants' of conventional theory, the Critical Theorist is conscious of their location within broader, physical and metaphysical social and knowledge systems, and is aware that their intellectual contribution seeks an explicit objective praxis *qua* social change. To this end Horkheimer stressed that Critical Theory should be 'neither "deeply rooted" like totalitarian propaganda nor "detached" like the liberal intelligentsia' (Horkheimer, 1982: 223-4). Such an 'inside/outside' duality was to be furthered through a flexible, interdisciplinary research programme, with an eliding, shifting focus, while remaining concerned with rationality and the ideological obfuscations of objective structural logics (Bronner, 2002, 2011). In this regard, Critical Theorists are thus most clearly unified by the themes of their research, and their political investment in an emancipatory rational society, rather than their application of research methodologies (Guess, 2004). Critical political economists such as Pollock and Grossman, and Critical legal scholars such as Neumann and Kirchheimer, worked on highly disparate research subjects, yet were united by the broader critique of social irrationality and by identifying the possibilities for immanent-transcendence. This interdisciplinary edge was further sharpened by Marcuse and Fromm who brought the left-Hegelian-Marxian sociological-philosophical approach into dialogue with social psychology and Freudian psychoanalysis (Delanty, 2011: 71-2).

There are two further themes central to the Critical Theoretical project, which partially unite the otherwise disparate cadre of quasi-Marxian academics: an explicit critique of the dominance of instrumental reason (Schecter, 2010) and a methodologically avowed anti-positivism (Osborne and Dews, 1987; Held, 2013). While both of these methodological and research interests are to some extent derivative of the German Idealist roots of the research project (Rush, 2013: 188), they continue to lead to the identification of new areas of social research. For example, today the critique of instrumental rationality is increasingly informing the Critical Digital Humanities (Berry, 2014; Fuchs, 2018).

While 'Third' and 'Fourth' generations of Critical Theory have moved away from their left-Hegelian foundations and explicitly embraced Apelian pragmatics and analytic philosophy (Frega, 2014), the focus on diagnosing social pathologies remains a central unifying concern across Frankfurt School scholarship (Honneth, 2007b; Chapter One). The framing of 'social pathology' is perhaps uniquely potent in that it captures both the distorting effects of ideology and the 'objective social problems' that ideology serves to obscure (Strydom, 2011). With this powerful dual purchase, 'social pathology' serves as both a highly efficient signifier, and a potent conceptual lens, through which Critical Theorists can identify the maladies of the social world.

Why research social pathology now?

With the ascendancy of increasingly restrictive, intersubjective approaches to social theory, the left-Hegelian-Marxian radicalism of earlier generations of Critical Theory is waning (Thompson, 2016). This has drastically impeded the Critical Theoretical diagnosis of social pathologies. As introduced above, Michael J. Thompson's (2016) polemic has catalysed a broader discussion on the 'domestication' of the Critical Theoretical project, which has divided the academy. Few would deny that Critical Theory has changed substantially in both its social-theoretical and political inflections over the last three decades. Siding with Thompson, I argue that recent developments in Critical Theory have marked a retreat from a direct confrontation with the primary source of social domination: the logics and rationalities central to capitalism. Accordingly, contemporary Critical Theory no longer informs progressive scholarship more broadly as it did in previous generations.[2] With increasingly contested philosophical foundations (critiqued as neo-Idealist) and an ever-closer alliance with capitalist norms and institutions,[3] Third (and Fourth)[4] generation Critical Theory is in a profound identity crisis. These tendencies can be evinced *tout court* through recent developments in social pathology scholarship.

While completing this thesis I was privileged to be a guest editor of a *European Journal of Social Theory* special issue on social pathologies and recognition. The contributions to the issue demonstrate both the timeliness of this research and the increasing polarisation of the debate. While papers from Thompson (2019) and Canivez (2019) served to further problematise the turn to recognition theoretical approaches to social pathology scholarship, various contributions served to extend the recognition approach, entirely oblivious to, or wilfully not engaging with, these increasingly prevalent critiques. Schaub and Odigbo (2019) evidence the drive to further radicalise the recognition approach, submitting that even the hunger of those waiting at foodbanks is best-theorised as an outcome of consumptive need misrecognition. Their paper made no acknowledgement that there is a mountainous literature opposing restrictive recognition-theoretical scholarship. To those critical of solely recognition approaches, such a

---

[2] For example, neither Wolfgang Streeck's *How Will Capitalism End*, nor Thomas Piketty's *Capital in the Twenty-First Century* draw extensively on contemporary Critical Theory.
[3] See Chapter One of Thompson's (2016) *The Domestication of Critical Theory*.
[4] Third and fourth generation Critical Theory exist contemporaneously. While Forst's appeal continues to grow, Honneth's recognition-derived approach has achieved such dominance, within and beyond Critical Theory, that his account remains the central paradigm for critical social theory.

framing may seem dogmatically wedded to the intersubjective paradigm, serving little to no explanatory value (McNay, 2006; Thompson, 2016). This is not to flag the co-authors Schaub and Odigbo for special criticism: on the contrary, this example is given as it is highly indicative of the debate more broadly. While the special issue was a success in bringing competing approaches to social pathology diagnosis within a singular volume, the edition indicates the increasingly siloed nature of the debate. In part, my seventh chapter serves as a response to the collected articles: showing how an 'inverted', radically reshaped, recognition paradigm could potentially be of some limited use as part of a broader Critical Theoretical approach.

In short, there is a battle raging in Critical Theory. For Michael J. Thompson, destabilising the hegemony of the neo-Idealist paradigm is an essential first-step in rejuvenating the Critical Theory tradition. My distinctive contribution is to focus explicitly on how pathology diagnosing critique has been impeded by the restrictive, neo-Idealist recognition-turn. By drawing out the artificial constraints of the recognition-derived approach to social pathology scholarship, and by highlighting the efficacy of displaced framings of pathology diagnosing social critique, this thesis responds to Thompson's call to challenge the domesticated state of contemporary Critical Theory while extending Thompson's scholarship through a new focus on pathology diagnosis and a targeted critique of recognition theory.[5]

On the Nature and Scope of this Project

What this thesis seeks to demonstrate

In its current form as a doctoral thesis this project is sharply restricted to 80,000 words, so must make an incisive, targeted intervention. I thus outline exactly what the project seeks to achieve, and perhaps more importantly, what has been deliberately excluded from consideration, while held ripe for further study.

While Critical Theory is, by definition, interdisciplinary, and this thesis draws upon aspects of intellectual history, gender theory, philosophy, political economy and psychoanalytic theory, this is ultimately a submission in social theory. The departures into other subject areas are thus excursions to further the two central social theoretical points of this thesis, which are:

    a) That the dominant form of recognition-derived social pathology scholarship is both social-theoretically restrictive and philosophically untenable and,

---

[5] Thompson's critique of the neo-Idealist tendencies of contemporary critical theory focuses on both Habermasian and Honnethian Critical Theory (as well as, to a lesser extent, Forst, *inter alia*). This project does not engage extensively with Habermas. My focus is on more contemporary debates, and thus the neo-Idealist tendencies in Honneth's work are afforded greater scrutiny.

b) That a plurality of potent, yet currently side-lined approaches for conducting social pathology diagnosis are lying dormant, due to the near total hegemony of recognition derived framings.

While the first submission is relatively self-contained in terms of the necessary content, the second was substantially more open-ended. While I ultimately opted to champion the breadth of social pathology diagnosing approaches proffered by Rousseau (Chapter Four), the pathologies of reason approach most associated with left-Hegelianism (Chapter Five), and the under-appreciated pathologies of normalcy approach presented by Erich Fromm (Chapter Six), I could just as readily explored the work of Jürgen Habermas, Theodore Adorno, Sigmund Freud or Walter Benjamin, *inter alia*. Equally, there could have been an entire chapter dedicated to Michael J. Thompson, or Axel Honneth. While it proved impossible within the constraints of a doctoral thesis to engage in the desired detail with the breadth of theorists who make important contributions to the discussion, the above all appear briefly and tangentially if not in more substantive analysis.

What this project is not

As a work of social theory, this project does not approach the study of social pathology from an explicitly philosophical angle, therefore many of the central concerns in the philosophical study of social pathology are absent. For example, there is only a limited discussion, in Chapter One, on the debates surrounding social organicism. Similarly, there is limited to no discussion on the growing literature on Dewey's insights for social pathology scholarship through his approach to 'social life' (Laitinen and Särkelä, 2019). Neither is there space for engaging with the extended philosophical literature on the classical origins of social pathology in Plato and Aristotle. Equally, this project does not seek to intervene in the debates around Antonovsky's (1996) conception of salutogenesis.[6]

While these concerns are of great interest and may have been central to any philosophical project engaging with social pathology scholarship, this thesis approaches Critical Theoretical scholarship from an explicitly social-theoretical perspective. While the above concerns would be of importance to a research project with a more pronounced philosophical inflection, they are not sufficiently proximate to my submission to merit inclusion herewith.

---

[6] Antonovsky's work originated within the field of medical sociology. In contrast to pathogenesis, which focuses on the factors that cause disease, salutogenesis focuses on factors that support human health and wellbeing. There is a growing scholarship which seeks to balance the two concerns (Mittelmark, 2016).

Finally, I wish to comment on the decision not to engage with Smith's (2017) *Society and Social Pathology,* which, *prima facie* would appear important for this project. While Smith's book is to be championed for its commitment to rigorous interdisciplinarity and for its rich incorporation of both qualitative and quantitative data, the project sits too far from both critical social theory and the current Frankfurt School debates on social pathology for it to feature within this strictly limited project. Smith's analysis is too distant from the politically potent debates surrounding social pathology and sits largely as a collection of interesting secondary textual analyses. There is little-to-no engagement with the dominant debates and literatures which the rest of this project situates itself. This is not to state that Smith's text is not worthy of further analysis, but will, due to limitations of space, have to wait along with the provocations on social pathology within the works of Habermas, Antonosky and Davis, for a future project.

Structure and Content

Beyond this introduction, the thesis consists of seven chapters and an extended conclusion.

Chapter One: *Social Pathology Diagnosis and Recognition: Very Different Beasts*

My opening chapter lays the foundations for the broader project by interrogating the central assumptions implicit in the thesis. It commences with a critical discussion of the merits of social pathology scholarship, framed through a brief historical sketch. While this theme is considered throughout the project, this first chapter offers a clear, non-partisan framing through which to conceptualise the approach more broadly. Having done so, the chapter then argues that pathology diagnosing social critique is philosophically justifiable and carries significant explanatory potential. The distinctive importance of social pathology diagnosis to the Critical Theory tradition is then elaborated. I then outline the approaches' distinctiveness from recognition theory. The second section of this chapter outlines how recognition has its own distinct heritage in social theory and philosophy and has no essential commonality with pathology diagnosing social critique. Honneth's radicalisation of recognition is introduced, while its continuing divergence from the core themes of pathology diagnosing critique is underscored.

Chapter Two: *Honneth's Critical Theory of Recognition: A Critique*

The second chapter outlines the political, philosophical and social-theoretical limitations of the dominant Honnethian recognition approach, which has come to impede social pathology scholarship. This chapter introduces the work of Michael J. Thompson (2016, 2019) and brings his critique of neo-Idealism into dialogue with Nancy Fraser's (2011) and Lois McNay's (2008) existing critiques of Honneth's recognition theory. As returned to in Chapter Seven, I argue here that the dominant recognition framing has substantial weaknesses and that without fundamental ontological and political changes this approach is best exercised from Critical Theoretical scholarship. Through the acritical return to the noumenal-idealist realm as the originary site of the social world (Bollenbeck, forthcoming), restrictive recognition theorists have negated Marx's (1961) foundational Copernican insight: that social existence precedes, and substantially determines, consciousness, which crucially impacts upon subjects' capacities to, and proclivities for, engagement in recognition relationships.

Chapter Three: *Recognition Theory and Social Pathology: A Troubling Marriage*

This third chapter charts how contemporary social pathology theorists have embraced Honneth's Critical Theory of Recognition. I outline how such a move has been furthered through the Jyväskylä's School's embrace of Honneth's scholarship (1995, 2008, 2014a, 2014b) and by Christoper Zurn's (2011) influential 'second-order' reading of Honneth's work. Extending Freyenhagen, I argue that both Zurn and Honneth are responsible for social pathologies increasingly being theorised as existing *solely* 'in the head' of the subject (Freyenhagen, 2015: 44), at variance with the broader Critical Theory tradition (Delanty, 2011; Strydom, 2011). The chapter then problematises Honneth's (2014) framing of 'misdevelopments', which is held to trap pathology diagnosis within the recognition register and further expedites Critical Theory's retreat from a direct engagement with capitalist logics and irrationalities. This chapter seeks to expose the problematically restrictive nature of the dominant, Honneth-Zurn inspired approach to social pathology scholarship. A section from of this chapter (between 1500-2000 words) has was published in the *European Journal of Social Theory* during the course of this research.

Chapter Four: Rousseau: The Social Pathologist *Par Excellence*

Having assessed the dominant recognition approach to social pathology scholarship (Chapters Two and Three), the following three chapters reconstruct alternate approaches to pathology diagnosing critique which have been needlessly displaced by the recognition paradigm. The first of these chapters, Chapter Four, engages with Rousseau's *oeuvre complète*. Five distinct framings of social pathology are located within Rousseau work. While Neuhouser (2012) has demonstrated the centrality of pathology diagnosis to Rousseau's *Discourse on Political Economy* (1758), this chapter engages with Rousseau's work as a totality, identifying penetrating forms of pathology diagnosing critique across his autobiography, his operas, his pedagogy and his musicology, in addition to his political economy and foundational social theory.[7] It is particularly gratifying to discover a plethora of framings of social pathology within Rousseau's work which are incompatible with the recognition account. That the recognition theorist *par excellence* transcended the recognition register to present his social critique is a telling indictment of the shockingly myopic nature of contemporary recognition-derived Critical Theory.

Chapter Five: *The Pathologies of Reason: Left-Hegelianism and Social Pathology*

Chapter Five focuses on the left-Hegelian tradition and the competing framings of 'pathologies of Reason' circulating within the broader critical discussion. While for Honneth (2004: 338), it is the left-Hegelian critique of deficient (cognitive and socially manifest) rationality which constitutes the 'explosive charge' of Critical Theory, the accompanying literature is formidably complicated (Marcuse, 1969). What is held to constitute a pathology of reason is increasingly contested (Honneth, 2007a). This chapter thus seeks to achieve three objectives: (a) to reconstruct the dominant understandings of pathologies of reason in circulation and to draw out their essential commonalities, (b) to demonstrate how these insights are of utility for Critical Theory, and, (c) to identify how these resources are needlessly excluded by the dominant recognition-derived approach to Critical Theory.

Chapter Six: *Reconstructing Erich Fromm's 'pathology of normalcy'*

While Fromm does not offer a singular text outlining a clear vision of social pathology, through engaging closely with his output one can reconstruct a sophisticated understanding of social pathology based on the economic and psycho-social mechanisms which serve to perpetuate the pathologies of the present. For Fromm (1963, 1983, 2010), the challenge is to expose how social pathologies are normalised, how subjects come to accept the 'insanity' of the social world. This chapter seeks to rehabilitate Fromm's approach to social pathology diagnosis and aims to show how his valuable insights are needlessly excluded by the dominant recognition paradigm to the detriment of Critical Theory.

---

[7] Situating Rousseau's project within such contemporary subject demarcations is of course anachronistic, and is therefore done apologetically, solely for its explanatory merit as a convenient typology.

Chapter Seven: *Rethinking Recognition*

Drawing out of the preceding three chapters, an inverted recognition approach is presented as a possible contribution to a future, broader, 'polycentric' social pathology diagnosing approach (Fraser and Honneth, 2001). Crucially, for recognition to play any such role, recognition-theorists' claims to the ontological primacy of the intersubjective dyad would need to be discarded, as would any argument in favour of a monistic social theory. In contrast to the hegemonic 'pathologies of recognition' framing, I contend that utilising a more nuanced recognition perspective could be useful as one route amongst many for exposing the full breadth of social pathologies. In my suggested, inverted recognition engagement, a focus on recognition relationships is of possible utility as a means of exposing some of the deeper social pathologies which exist *beyond* the recognition register. This submission is offered as a means of retaining the insights of recognition theory, while transcending the needlessly restrictive and philosophically problematic foundations of the dominant recognition-monist approach. I stress that my suggested re-imagining of recognition exists as one amongst many approaches for exposing and conceptualising the pathologies of the social world. In part it is offered to start bridging the chasm between Honnethian recognition theorists and those who retain a stronger investment in a polycentric and dialectical Marxian Critical Theory.

Conclusion: *Social Pathology Diagnosis and the Future of Critical Theory*

The thesis finishes with an extended conclusion. My central social-theoretical submission is reasserted within a discussion of broader debates in contemporary Critical Theory. I present this thesis as a contribution towards the critique of domesticated, contemporary 'Third' and 'Fourth' generation Critical Theory. My social theoretical submission is then positioned relative to its future possible application for social research. The final lines speak of the importance of having rigorous, polycentric pathology diagnosing foundations for future Critical Theoretical scholarship.

A Final Consideration

Critical Theorists diagnose social pathologies to advance the progressive transformation of the irrational social order. This thesis sits as part of the broader campaign to renew the radicalism of the Critical Theory tradition, and to reinvigorate the political-transformative objectives of the broader research project. As this thesis will submit, Honneth's Critical Theory of Recognition is a clear impediment to this objective. Instead of focusing on the objective contradictions in the capitalist social world, and the ideological artifice that obscures them, Honnethian Critical Theory focuses on developing ever more ingenious ways to convince social subjects that capitalist society already offers the potential for emancipation and a flourishing existence (Honneth, 2014b: 8, 46). In *Freedom's Right* (2014), Honneth substituted the immanent-transcendent methodology, with its appreciation of Hegelian latency, for a metaphysically absent conservative presentism. The dominant approach to social pathologies is unjustifiable: social pathologies are not solely located 'in the head' of the subject, rather there are irrationalities within the objective social order which require incisive theoretical analysis and urgent political transformation (Strydom, 2011). The diagnosis of social pathologies has long offered a crucial tool to engage in deeper, more penetrating social critique; a means of looking beyond the dominant social mores and to expose contradictory social logics (Honneth, 2004). By reasserting the critical potential of the pathology diagnosing tradition, which ironically Honneth (2000, 2003, 2004a, 2007a, 2007b, 2007c, 2014a) himself has outlined better than anybody, I hope Critical Theorists can once again point towards the more rational society latent within the contradictions of today's capitalist social conjecture (Delanty, 2011; Strydom, 2011).

Chapter One

Social Pathology Diagnosis and Recognition: Very Different Beasts

Introduction

This thesis argues that the diagnosis of social pathologies is rapidly being rendered impotent through its troubling marriage with Honneth's restrictive recognition approach to social theory. But when one steps back for the shortest moment it is immediately apparent that this submission is loaded with assumptions which require interrogation. This first chapter seeks to do just that, to lay the foundations for the broader thesis by investigating the theoretical commitments which undergird the central argument. This chapter thus engages with integral questions such as: What is social pathology diagnosis and is it something worth saving? Is social pathology diagnosis central to Critical Theory? Isn't the language of 'pathology' problematic in itself? In today's conditions of normative crisis can we even state that society has pathologies with any certainty? Equally, what is meant by 'recognition'? Perhaps both 'social pathology' and 'recognition' share some foundational theoretical assumptions or insights, therefore their increasing fusion in the literature is not merely contingent and undesirable, but positive and/or inevitable? How is Honneth's approach to recognition distinct from the understandings of recognition which preceded it?

This chapter engages with these questions by outlining the distinct historical development of social pathology diagnosis and recognition. The central argument flowing through this chapter is that recognition and social pathology offer fundamentally divergent approaches to study the social world: they help develop different knowledge interests and have distinct philosophical and social-theoretical foundations.

The chapter is divided into two sections. First, by drawing on Honneth (2000, 2004a, 2007a, 2007b, 2007c, 2014a *inter alia*) and Neuhouser (2012), I argue for the distinctive importance of social pathology diagnosing critique for Critical Theory. This section outlines the development of social pathology scholarship from its ancient origins in Plato to Honneth's contemporary analyses, and demonstrates the complex tapestry of ideas that converged in its Critical Theoretical genealogy (Honneth, 2007a). I then engage with concerns stemming from the biological language and framing of 'pathology', and the philosophical question of how one can conduct such explicitly normative critique in today's conditions of normative crisis (Honneth, 2004a, 2007b). Through outlining the *incidental* nature of the medicalised language, and the theoretical potency and philosophical justifiability of the approach, this section seeks to justify my investment in social pathology diagnosing critique.

The second section focuses on recognition. Through charting the development of recognition as a social-theoretical construct, I outline its distinctive features and further differentiate the framing from social pathology diagnosing critique. I argue that while recognition has proved of tremendous import to social theory for centuries, recent developments have led to a radical reimagining of the framework. Through outlining the distinctive development of Honneth's Critical Theory of Recognition, the final part of this section argues that while Honneth has reoriented both recognition and Critical Theory, 'recognition' remains an entirely distinct framework to social pathology. The origins of Honneth's recognition approach are presented, serving as an introduction to his importance for this project more broadly.

This first chapter thus lays the necessary foundations for my core submission. As stated in my introduction, this thesis marks a distinctly critical engagement with Honnethian recognition-derived approaches to social pathology scholarship (how he 'does' social pathology diagnosis). Yet, equally, I draw heavily upon Honneth's analysis of the social pathology tradition (how Honneth 'gets' the importance of social pathology). This contradictory relationship with Honneth's work continues throughout the project.

Pathology diagnosis: the history and utility of a central resource for Critical Theory

Critical Theory and the Syncretic Nature of Social Pathology Diagnosis

Whitehead famously declared that Western philosophy[8] 'consists of a series of footnotes to Plato' (Whitehead, 1979: 39). It should thus perhaps come as little surprise then, that the first engagement with a framing of societal malfunctioning, or societal illness, can be found in *The Republic* (Plato, 2008: 369a-372d). During Socrates'[9] discussion of the 'City of Pigs', the hypostatized pastoral idyll of a city, Socrates warns that the 'polis' can enter a 'fevered state' when 'unnatural desires' for luxury goods come to dominate (Plato, 2008: 369a-372d). Such problematic luxury is presented as a harmful deviation from the pastoral; typified by the excessive consumption of alcohol, or of fatty sauces (Plato, 2008: 372c). It is a little unclear whether the prevalence of these 'unnatural desires' constitutes a 'fever' in itself, or if the distinctly 'fevered' quality arises only when a particular dynamic is precipitated. Wealth is sought

---

[8] Of course, there are many discussions on topics similar to 'social pathology' in non-Western social-theory and social-philosophy. Consider, for instance, Jiddu Krishnamurti's (2008) work on the question of adjustment to alienating social norms. The core message Krishnamurti offered to his followers was 'it is no measure of health to adjust oneself to an unwell society', this sounds remarkably similar to Fromm's engagement with social pathology. However, due to my investment in the Critical Theoretical tradition, combined with the restrictive nature of a doctoral thesis, these approaches will have to wait for a future project.

[9] As ever, it is unclear to what extent Socrates functions as a 'mouth-piece' for Plato, or whether this is an accurate representation of Socrates' own position (Cohn, 2001).

to determine one's status, yet such status determination can occur only relationally (Plato, 2008: 373a). Thus the 'fevered' society exhibits the following dynamic of negative infinity: ever greater luxury is sought to show a relationally higher standing, leading to an insatiable acquisitive drive. This dynamic has no determinable end, and risks exhausting all social resources. For Plato, it appears to be *society itself* that is 'fevered' (Plato, 2008: 373a). In the spirit of Whitehead's axiom, Neuhouser has connected Plato's discussion of fevered societies to Rousseau's analysis of 'amour-propre' two millennia later (Neuhouser, 2012). For Neuhouser, the focus on negative dynamics remains crucially important to ideas of social pathology diagnosis today (Neuhouser, 2012: 631). Plato marks an early contribution to a distinct species of social criticism that utilises the language, and structure, of the diagnosis of societal illnesses, and attendant impaired functionality.

Following his tutor's lead, Aristotle's *Politics* utilises similar framings. Commentators have suggested that *Politics* can be read as a diagnosis of 'political pathology' (Tracy, 1969: 304). Aristotle's use of the norm of health when determining the 'proportionate blend' of the 'mixed constitution' continues this approach, but in a subtly different vein (Aristotle, 2009: 1302b33-1303a3). As with Plato, it is society itself that can exhibit 'pathologies', not (necessarily) the social subjects. Society is again discussed, albeit analogously, as a corporeal meta-subject, presaging the weak social organicism of the Frankfurt School tradition (Strydom, 2011). From Plato to Aristotle, to the Scholasticism that gripped Europe, social criticism has a long tradition of turning to the language of the bodily to critique impaired social functioning (Nájera, 2017). In his extensive discussions on social pathology diagnosis, Honneth charts a similar genesis (Honneth, 2007c). In continuing accord with Honneth, I contend that despite its millennia of history, the pathology diagnosing approach only attained maturity with the writings of Rousseau in the eighteenth century (Honneth, 2007c: 5).

The scholarly orthodoxy is to pose a division in Rousseau's works between efforts to diagnose social pathologies and attempted remedies (Wokler, 2001; Chapter Four). The *Discourse on Political Economy*, the *Discourse on the Arts and the Sciences* ('The First Discourse'), and the *Discourse on the Origins of Inequality* ('The Second Discourse'), are often read as the 'diagnosis', while *The Social Contract* and *Emile* are often presented as the 'cure'. It is with the *Discourses* that the tradition of social pathology diagnosing critique developed in earnest. For Honneth, Rousseau's polemical social critique is significant for it represented a rejection 'of an entire form of life' (Honneth, 2007c: 7), rather than a 'mere investigation of ... political-moral legitimacy (Honneth, 2007c: 10). The focus of Rousseau's investigation was 'the structural limitations ... (society) imposes on the goal of human self-realization' (Honneth, 2007c: 10), an examination of the obstacles to subjects attaining the good life. It is this change in focus, a move away from analyses of injustice or illegitimacy, and towards an analysis of the societal flaws preventing subjects achieving self-realization, which marks the true maturation of social pathology diagnosing critique as a form of social criticism *sui generis*.

It is perhaps the 'Second Discourse' which reads most evidently as a critique of the development of modern civilisation. Here, the *citoyen de Geneve* iconoclastically declares that man is 'naturally good' (Rousseau, 1984: 147), yet 'the extreme inequalities of our ways of life' make us 'wretched' (Rousseau, 1984: 84). There is nothing natural to:

> The excess of idleness among some and the excess of toil among others, the ease of stimulating and gratifying our appetites and our senses, the over-elaborate foods of the rich, which inflame and overwhelm them with indigestion, the bad food of the poor, which they often go without altogether, so that they over-eat greedily when they have the opportunity; those late nights, excesses of all kinds, immoderate transports of every passion, fatigue, exhaustion of mind, the innumerable sorrows and anxieties that people in all classes suffer, and by which the human soul is constantly tormented: these are the fatal proofs that most of our ills are of our own making, and that we might have avoided nearly all of them if we had adhered to the simple, unchanging and solitary way of life that nature ordained for us (Rousseau, 1984: 84-85).

Rousseau argued that 'vanity and scorn' (Rousseau, 1984: 114) were the hallmarks of civilisation. Such vices are presented as anathema to 'natural man', who lived in a 'golden mean' 'between the indolence of the primitive state and the petulant activity of our own pride' (Rousseau, 1984: 115). Rousseau's philosophy represents a critique of foundational social developments which inhibit the capacity of man to achieve a good and happy life. For Neuhouser, it is the profundity of this critique, the depth of the deviation from the social conditions necessary for subjects' self-actualisation, that makes Rousseau the social pathologist *par excellence* (Neuhouser, 2012).

With Rousseau, social pathology diagnosis developed into a critique of the direction society had taken in its entirety, directly confronting a world where man was 'born free, yet everywhere he is in chains' (Rousseau, 1968: 49). For Rousseau such a society was making man both physically ill and chronically restricting his capacity for self-realisation. In one intriguing passage Rousseau comments, 'we could write the history of human illness by following the history of civilized societies' (Rousseau, 1984: 85); yet, this fascinating contention aside, Rousseau's diagnosis is of wretchedness more than biological ill health. Rousseau perhaps marks the zenith of pathology diagnosing social critique which submits that society itself may be suffering from its own faults and flaws, and that its sub-optimal functioning inhibits the capacity of its members to attain self-realisation.

With the Frankfurt School, social pathology diagnosis came to bridge the diagnostic endeavour of Rousseau, introduced above, with a species of critique developed by Hegel. Hegel brought forward a radicalisation of the critique of reason (Marcuse, 1969); framing rationality both as a social product, and as a metaphysical layer of the socio-political (Dahbour, 2017: 87-108). Reason for Hegel, in Marcuse's words, was more 'task' and less 'fact' (Marcuse, 1969). This radicalisation of the critique of reason remains a crucial aspect of Critical Theory (Held, 2013). As Honneth submits, 'that social pathologies are to be understood as a result of deficient rationality is ultimately indebted to the political philosophy of Hegel' (Honneth, 2004a: 341). For the first generation of Frankfurt School scholars, it was the Hegelian framing of 'historically effective reason' that centred their Critical Theory (Honneth, 2004a). Crudely summarising Hegel's sophisticated socio-political philosophy, one can say: it is only when society lives up to the highest standard of reason that it is capable of maintaining that social subjects will live good and happy lives. Thus, left-Hegelians broadly strive for a 'rational' society, critiquing the aspects of social life which fail to live up to the highest possible existing standard of reason (Marcuse, 1969). The species of pathology diagnosing critique adopted by Critical Theory imbibes Hegel's critique of reason, adding an essential second lens to its optics. One can already see how social pathology diagnosis presents as a multi-layered theoretical endeavour: building on the Rousseauian diagnosis of society as inhibiting the capacity of subjects to achieve self-realisation, with the Hegelian critique of societal irrationality. The social institutions and processes that inhibit self-realisation are thus framed as evincing deficient social rationality. Rationality is manifest, and perpetuated, both socially, and in cognitive form: in the subjects themselves. Thus, the Critical Theoretical diagnosis of social pathologies focuses on both the social institutions themselves, and the ideological artifice that maintains them through the cognitive impairments induced in the social subjects (Strydom, 2011; Held, 2013).

Following Hegel, left-Hegelian thought centres a similar critique of rationality. As Honneth contends, in their various formulations, left-Hegelians submit that 'a rational universal is always required for the possibility of fulfilled self-realization within society' (Honneth, 2004a: 341). The 'rational universal' refers to the idea expressed above, that the highest possible standard of socially existing reason needs to be operative throughout the contours of social life. Within varying objects of critique: the market, the family etc, the desire for a 'rational praxis' (this optimal rationality manifesting in the social world) remains a constant. For Marx, for instance, the 'social pathology' is that 'the actual organisation of society …. [falls] short of the standards of rationality that are already embedded in the forces of production' (Honneth, 2004a: 340). Synthesising Rousseau's understanding of pathology diagnosis with Hegel's, one can read (with crude simplification) the central Marxist critique, as a species of pathology diagnosis thus: the actual organisation of society, in the capitalist political economy, does not live up to the highest standards of rationality that already exist, this sub-optimal social functioning prevents social subjects from attaining the good life. A more rational, post-capitalist society lies latent within the irrational present.[10]

Another layer of analysis is added with the incorporation of the psychoanalytic dimension to social pathology diagnosis. Freud, and the lesser known Mitscherlich, both mark important developments to pathology diagnosing critique (Honneth, 2014a). Freud (1953) analysed the explicitly 'social neuroses', these repressive social dynamics that produce anxious and neurotic subjects. Freud depicts society, as a meta-subject, suffering from 'neuroses'; thus, producing unwell citizens. That society can be structured in such a way to create neurotic subjects adds an additional psychoanalytic layer to the pathology diagnosing endeavour. When society 'habituate(s) … situations and conditions of satisfaction that are not normal', the 'most obvious outcome is nervous illness' (Freud, 1959: 201-2). It is worth stressing that for Freud, with a clear implicit ontological assumption about the social body: both society and the social subjects are unwell.[11] In many ways this style of social pathology diagnosis overlaps with Rousseau's: social actors are suffering because society is constructed in ways that oppose the subjects achieving self-actualisation. Learning from Freud and Mitscherlich, Critical Theorists incorporated an analysis of how the distorted social rationality impacts subjects at a psychoanalytic register.

One important aspect of both the Freudian and Mitscherlichian approach is that the suffering of society's members, as a result of the deformed state is reason, is framed medically, and restricted to the clinically unwell. Rather than the 'chained' and 'wretched' (Rousseau, 1968) of Rousseau, it is a discussion of the 'neurotic' and 'ill' (Freud, 1959) for Freud and Mitscherlich. It should be noted that while Critical Theory draws extensively on psychoanalysis to diagnose societal irrationalities, it does not follow the contention that a social pathology requires medically 'ill' subjects (Honneth, 2014a: 698). Rather, drawing from Freud, Critical Theorists 'establish a connection between defective rationality and individual suffering' at a psychological level (Honneth, 2007c: 38) and are thus able to immanently ground their critique of reason. Deficient social rationality is experienced in psychic suffering in the social subject through neuroses and alienation more broadly, not merely through clinical diagnosis. Thus, Critical Theorists do not seek to connect manifest social irrationalities to symptoms present within the DSM (for example): the connection to the immanent is more holistic.

---

[10] Benjamin is distinct amongst Critical Theorists in viewing the latency of the more rational future to be most accessible through a speculative cultural history, yet even his account retains the core idea that the possibilities for a better future remain dormant and extant, even if it kept alive through the memory of the past resonating in the cultural present (Caygill, 2004).

[11] One can read the 'strong naturalism' of this account being distinct from the 'weak naturalism' of Critical Theory more broadly (Strydom, 2011).

With origins in *The Republic*, reaching maturity with Rousseau, adding essential timbre with Hegel's critique of historically effective reason, and drawing on the insights of psychoanalysis, the diagnosis of social pathologies became 'the distinctive theoretical resource of Critical Theory' (Freyenhagen, 2015: 131). Drawing strongly on its left-Hegelian roots, it was the diagnosis of the pathological deviation of rationality under capitalism that gave Critical Theory its 'explosive charge' (Honneth, 2004a: 338). As framed in my introduction, Critical Theory engaged these irrationalities through a consciously interdisciplinary project; drawing upon the methodologies of political-economy, psychoanalysis, psychology, philosophy and legal theory (Held, 2013; Jeffries, 2017).

Horkheimer and Adorno's *Dialectic of Enlightenment* (1944) has been presented as the diagnosis of social pathology *par excellence* (Honneth, 2000). In this text, Adorno and Horkheimer obliquely disclose how a species of reason, *instrumental rationality*, has come to dominate human thought, with devastating effects (Roberts, 2004). Their highly idiosyncratic work is read by Honneth as a presentation that the existing 'social circumstances violates those conditions which constitute a necessary presupposition for a good life amongst us' (Honneth, 2000: 122). In *Dialectic of Enlightenment* the social pathology is primarily one of a deformed rationality which has developed an 'extraordinary sweep' (Adorno and Horkheimer, 1997: 61), through which subjects fail to grasp the particularities of the life-world, instead perceiving 'the particular only as one case of the general' (Adorno and Horkheimer, 1997: 84-5). This foundational epistemic corruption is considered a crucial antecedent for the 'new kind(s) of barbarism' of late capitalism (Adorno and Horkheimer: xi). *Dialectic of Enlightenment* is a highly idiosyncratic text, and the presentation and structure of the work makes engagement challenging. However, the authors' ambition to disclose the incompatibility of unalienated, meaningful existence, with an instrumental rationality run amok, remains central.

While *Dialectic of Enlightenment* constitutes a diagnosis of social pathology at a macrocosmic, epistemic, foundational level; works of Critical Theory have tended to represent a targeted engagement with instantiations of social irrationality. As stated, Critical Theory utilises a spectrum of disciplines to engage with the social (Held, 2013), and thus the framing of social pathology diagnosis has been adapted for divergent (inter-)disciplinary parameters.

The work of psychologist and psychoanalyst, Erich Fromm, for instance, represents a sustained engagement with social pathology drawing upon Marx and Freud (see Chapter Six). In an analysis which flows between texts, Fromm (1951) articulates the 'pathology of normalcy', how the inadequacies and irrationalities of the capitalist societies are perpetuated through their acceptance as 'normality' (Fromm, 2010). In *The Sane Society* (1963), Fromm epitomises how the pathology framing has been used to engage with both problematically irrational social arrangements (in the objective, manifest social world) and the ideological or cognitive impairments which inhibit social subjects from emancipation, and which impede progressive political praxis.

Similarly, the economist and political scientist, Friedrich Pollock (1928) articulates the irrationalities present in state-capitalist political-economies. Nancy Fraser's engagement with critical political economy continues this tradition today (Fraser and Jaeggi, 2018). The relationship between pathology diagnosis and negative dynamics in the work of both Pollock and Fraser returns my discussion to the earliest framing of social pathology as found in *The Republic*. Neuhouser's intellectual history has charted the diagnosis of social pathologies within the economic organisation of society back to Rousseau's *Discourse on Political Economy* and explores five distinct manifestations of the heuristic within that sole work (Neuhouser, 2012). Bonefeld's *Critical Theory and the Critique of Political Economy* (2014) offers yet another recent substantial Critical Theoretical engagement with political economy and social pathology. Bonefeld's more distanced relationship to the critique of pathologies of reason adds further nuance and timbre to pathology diagnosing critique.

The diagnosis of social pathologies is thus a Critical Theoretical constant; even within works that do not explicitly utilise pathology diagnosis as their central analytical resource. Marcuse, for instance, speaks of the 'pathological deformation' of the personality in *One Dimensional Man* (1964), while Habermas' *Reflections on Communicative Pathology* (2001) identifies the pathological deformations of the communicative realm. Neumann details the pathological anxieties arising from the atomistic foundations of 'democratic will formation' (Honneth, 2003). Even Adorno's *Minima Moralia* (1951), a work oft-cited as more poetic lament than social theory (van den Brink, 1997), retains the social pathology diagnosing rubric upon closer analysis (Honneth, 2004a). In a telling passage Adorno (1978) explicitly links the various facets of damaged life to the loss of a good universal, and thus fundamentally connects his analysis to the limitations precipitated by deficiencies in the historically existing societal rationality. It is as if Critical Theorists are unable to help themselves from diagnosing social pathologies: there is a driving force within the research project which pushes its practitioners to attempt to capture the essence of the social malady, to seek out the core contradictions of the social conjecture. It thus seems entirely justified to argue that an engagement with social pathology has been a constant thread throughout the Critical Theory tradition and one which can be charted in the key canonical literature which social theoretically and philosophically informs the project (Honneth, 2007c).

This first section has charted the development of a distinct species of critique: social pathology diagnosis. It has tracked the framing's origins in Ancient philosophy, articulated the importance of Rousseau (see Chapter Four), Hegel (see Chapter Five) and Fromm (see Chapter Six), and discussed the centrality of the approach to first, second and third generation Frankfurt School Critical Theorists. This engagement has demonstrated the prevalence of the diagnosis of social pathologies over time 'as an alternative to the mainstream liberal' mode of critique (Freyenhagen, 2015: 131) and has outlined the complexity of its development. I have presented social pathology diagnosis as a valuable tool for analysing deformations in socially effective reason, and the precipitant impact on the capacity of subjects to attain self-realisation. This analysis has shown how pathology diagnosis today draws on a multiplicity of theorists, traditions and disciplines, including Rousseau (Chapter Four), Hegel (Chapter Five) and Fromm (Chapter Six).

Social Pathology Diagnosis: A social-theoretically and philosophically justifiable framework for social critique

Having established that the diagnosis of social pathologies represents the 'distinctive resource' (Freyenhagen, 2015; 131) of Critical Theory; I now subject the approach to detailed scrutiny. I start by problematising the strong naturalistic (or 'organismic') conception of society, which, *prima facie*, appears necessary for the diagnosis of such pathologies.[12] This discussion leads into questions of social functioning and the problems of philosophically justifying a species of critique built on an apparently partisan, and teleological understanding of society. Drawing on Honneth (2000, 2004a, 2007a, 2007b, 2007c, 2014a *inter alia*) and Neuhouser (2012), I contend that these challenges can be sufficiently addressed. Further, I argue that the optic of pathology diagnosis enables a crucial, 'thicker' species of social critique. I argue that through the exposition and analysis of socially defective reason, made possible through pathology diagnosing critique, 'forms of life' can be critically appraised. Social pathology diagnosis is thus positioned as an essential prerequisite for Critical Theory's 'deeper' engagement with the social.

On the signifier 'pathology' and the ontology of the signified

It is worth engaging directly with both the language and the idea of a biologically 'unhealthy' society. As discussed, Plato, Rousseau and Freud all expressly speak of society itself as 'fevered'

---

[12] As stated in my introduction, there is an interesting and growing philosophical literature on these concerns, however, due to the social-theoretical nature of this project, and limitations in space, I am unable to delve too far into these debates here.

or 'neurotic'. One might thus suspect that social pathology diagnosis necessitates a strong, exaggerated naturalism, presenting society as a living entity that can be studied and 'diagnosed' using the tools of the natural sciences. Following MacLay (1990), it might be submitted that social pathology diagnosis is based on a strong 'socially organismic' understanding. Such organicism attracts substantial criticism (Struve, 1978). Arguably it is a product of too 'fantastic an imagination'; representing an implicit ontological statement that cannot be justified philosophically (McGee, 1991). Such critiques contend that society plainly is 'not alive' as understood biologically; society simply is not 'an organism' in any meaningful way. Further, even if a philosophical justification could be found for comprehending society organismically, this would merely precipitate further serious, potentially irredeemable, complications. The 'organism' presented by society would be so wildly divergent to all organisms hitherto studied that it would require the creation of unique, and inevitably *political*, instruments of analysis.

Critics have further contended that the framing of 'objective biological illness' is both politically dangerous and academically anachronistic (Honneth, 2014a: 684). Discussions of 'degenerate societies', and 'healthier societies', have a sinister, and well charted history, for both the political right and left; sharing the semantic field of fascism, ethnic cleansing, and eugenics (Sewell, 2009). Further, following Foucault's (1963) *The Birth of the Clinic*, 'illness' and 'health' are now often understood as social constructs, created discursively, rather than bearing any unmediated relation to objective biological impairment (Foucault, 1963). For Foucault, the discourse of 'pathology' is utilised to bring forth subjectivities for 'disciplining' (Dreyfus and Rabinow, 1982: 173). In such an understanding, the language of 'the pathological', 'the sick' and 'the deviant', refers to discursively constructed categorisations, utilised to legitimate governmentality rather than to further emancipation (Foucault, 1963). The very idea that biologically framed social illness should function as an objective referent for social criticism thus appears academically destabilised and politically untenable.

Various rejoinders can be rallied. First, a distinction needs to be drawn between thinkers who explicitly embrace a strong naturalist ontology, and those who merely utilise the pathology framings for its explanatory utility while retaining a fidelity to the weak naturalism common to Critical Theory (Strydom, 2011; Honneth, 2014a). An obvious difference exists between arguing society is, *ontologically*, a living organism, and simply utilising such an organismic framing *analogously* to further one's argument (MacLay, 1990). The pathology diagnosing tradition has traditionally been read as reflecting the 'weak naturalism' of Critical Theory (Strydom, 2011: 10). I thus contend the species of pathology diagnosing critique deployed by Critical Theory is not essentially predicated on a 'strong' organismic understanding of the social. Rather, the inference is that,

> there is a continuity between nature and the socio-cultural form of life ... [a] relation .... [which] is not [to be] interpreted in a strong determinate sense which could lead to an epistemological reduction of society to nature (Strydom, 2011: 10).

Alternative arguments could also be submitted which negate the commitment to a weak naturalistic understanding of the social. As presented here, the core submission of a diagnosis of social pathology is that society is failing to function at its optimum capacity. There is no essential naturalism to the notion of functionality: one can speak of a functional helicopter as much as a functioning liver. From such a position one could argue that the usage of the biological analogy is just that, an analogy, and an alternate lexical framing, could, and quite possibly, *should*, be utilised; both to displace unhelpful incidental ontological critiques and to negate concerns over the language of 'pathology'. Indeed, it is undeniable that the lexicon of 'illness' brings with it political and academic complications. A more prudent framing would perhaps be to discard the language of 'pathology' and 'diagnosis' altogether, and instead utilise the explicit terminology of 'functionality' and 'impaired functionality'. The alternate analogy of a machine, impaired in its workings, could have similar utility, while avoiding some of the political complications with the analogy of illness.

The first rejoinder sought to embrace the language of the natural while rejecting the 'epistemological reduction of society to nature' (Strydom, 2011: 10). The second rejoinder claims that the language of the 'natural' and thereby of 'pathology' is merely incidental.

The second response, that the language of biological illness could, and arguably *should*, be rejected, and replaced with the language of 'impaired functionality', would fail to appease the challenges brought forth from a Foucauldian paradigm. The shift from 'illness' to 'impaired functionality', utilising a new mechanical analogy, could be understood as mere 'New Speak'. The state would simply bring forth subjectivities that could be 'legitimately disciplined' along these new terms of 'impaired functionality'. My second rejoinder is that Foucault's critique is of the impact of 'illness' and other such discursive markers *on subjects* (Foucault, 2003: especially Chapter Two). Social pathology diagnosis works at a different register, analysing society itself, as a totality. The 'diagnoses' and 'pathologies' of the social, articulated by Critical Theorists, refer to a 'form of life' (Honneth, 2000: 119; Jaeggi, 2018) and do not mark an engagement with subjects either as individuals, or as collective groups. The object of analysis is the social meta-subject. The framings of illness at this register cannot (at least in any proximate, immediate manner) legitimate the state's disciplining of subjects; indeed, often, in Critical Theoretical analysis, the state itself is the object of critique (Pollock, 1941, *inter alia*).

In response to the critiques that social pathology diagnosis has unavoidable foundations in social organicism, and brings forth a politically, and academically unsound framing of the social, multiple rejoinders have been offered (Honneth, 2004a). One can embrace a weak naturalism which has traditionally been the approach favoured by Critical Theorists (Strydom, 2011), yet other alternatives are equally justifiable. Social pathology diagnosis can be understood as making purely analogous use of the biological, rather than necessitating any strong ontological submission. The biological referent and language of social pathology is thus understood as merely incidental; indeed, shifting to the lexicon of mechanics might be pragmatic transition. In response to the Foucauldian caution against the lexicon of 'illness' and 'diagnosis', one can respond that social pathology diagnoses operates at a 'higher' register; focusing not on social subjects, but the entire subject of the social. Critical Theorists do not diagnose subjects as pathological; rather the diagnosis is of social dynamics and modalities more generally as evincing (a) defective form(s) of reason.

Normative Challenges

Even if one accepts that the signifier 'social pathology' is incidental, signifying the theorists' investment in 'deeper' problems of societal 'irrationality' or 'impeded functioning', various social-theoretical and philosophical questions arise. Does society even have a function or a deeper rationality? If so, how might theorists determine what it is? And how can social theorists justifiably talk of 'impaired social functioning' or 'societal irrationality' while these fundamental questions remain contested? Perhaps, most significantly, why would such a species of critique be of use? How would such a critique of 'social irrationality' or impeded functionality extend the tried and tested liberal framings of justice and legitimacy? Because first-generation Critical Theorists wrote before the post-structuralist and post-modernist assault on normativity they did not engage with such concerns (at least not explicitly, or in the same language). While there is no space in this project to engage with these topics in the detail required to do them justice, an abridged attempt follows below.

It might be submitted that any suggested societal 'function' or 'rational organisation' would necessarily be based on a partisan, teleological, understanding of society, which today seems, *prima facie*, normatively unjustifiable. Logically, it is impossible to diagnose society as 'irrational', 'non-functional', or 'impaired' in its functioning, without some referent to society's 'function' or transcendent sense of 'rationality'. Agreement about 'rationality' or 'functionality' thus appears to be imperative for this species of critique to be meaningful. While there remains no consensus on the conditions of an ideally rational or functional society, how can social theorists engage in such critique in a justifiable manner? With the ascent of post-modern and post-structuralist thought, variations on this normative concern have been challenging Critical Theory, and sociological theory more broadly, for the last forty years (Honneth, 2004a, 2014a).

Honneth (2000, 2004a, 2014a) has written extensively on the normative challenges posed to social theory and marks the most pronounced engagement with their implications for social pathology diagnosis. While acknowledging the severity of the normative challenge, Honneth does not attempt to produce a theoretical panacea. Instead, Honneth advances a working patch, of a 'weak formal anthropology', as a foundation for pathology diagnosing social critique (Honneth, 2007a). By turning to the foundational, anthropological needs of the human animal, Honneth submits that the social theorist can justifiably engage in discussion on 'formal conceptions of ethical life' (Honneth, 1995: 171-9). If one is 'sufficiently abstract' (Honneth, 2005: 174), the charge of partisanship, of 'embodying particular visions of the good life' will be unsustainable (Honneth, 1995: 174). The normative questions are neither 'solved' nor 'negated'. Instead, this weaker, formalistic understanding of the social enables discussion to take place with minimal norm-enshrining, and norm-dependant content. One can read Honneth's weak formal anthropology functioning as a meta-theoretical 'patch'; in this light he does not seek to solve the normative challenge; instead, he seeks to facilitate the conditions in which social theory can continue while such fundamental questions are further problematised.

Neuhouser offers a radically different response to the 'philosophical questions' that plague attempts at 'ascribing ends to social practices and institutions' (Neuhouser, 2012: 628-632). In contrast to Honneth, Neuhouser submits such squeamishness to ethical partisanship merely demarcates the perimeters of liberal thought (Neuhouser, 2012). In Neuhouser's work the reality of an ethical component to social critique is neither counter-productive nor philosophically problematic: it is merely seen an accepted facet of non-liberal social theory and social philosophy (Neuhouser, 2012). This embrace of ethical postulates is based on Neuhouser's submission that some commitment to 'conceptions of the good, or of human flourishing' is essential for critical thought that is 'thicker' than the limiting confines of 'liberal theories of justice' (Neuhouser, 2012: 628-632). For Neuhouser, there is no aporia here:

> A social theory that takes the idea of social pathology theory (seriously) rests implicitly on a vision of social reality according to which the social, as distinct from the merely political, cannot be adequately grasped or evaluated without attributing ends to social practices and institutions that are in a broad sense ethical (in the sense of being bound up with ideas of the good life or human flourishing)' (Neuhouser, 2012: 630).

For Neuhouser this is no cause for alarm; he considers the ethical embrace to be not a defect of the theoretical approach I am trying to articulate but a necessary consequence of the fact that what it takes as its object is social reality, not merely the political realm (Neuhouser, 2012: 630).

In Neuhouser's framing the appeal to social functionality is simply a reality of 'thick' social criticism and a result of the complexities of the social world. When one moves beyond the confines of liberal thought an imbrication in ethical postulates is inevitable, and reflects the complexities of the social, rather than a limitation of the approach to critique.

When one holds Honneth's and Neuhouser's submissions in tandem, a satisfactory rebuttal to the ethical challenge can easily be rallied. A critique of the social as 'irrational', or 'functionally impaired', can be justifiably built on a thin, formal anthropology. If this fails to appease the normative challenge, one could offer Neuhouser's rebuttal: 'thick' social criticism is based on the (partisan) attribution of ends to social practices. This is an existential reality of 'thick' social philosophy and is foundational for a deeper engagement with the social realm. Critical Theorists have long been aware of this fact. As stated in the introduction, Horkheimer's (1975) signal essay, 'Traditional and Critical Theory', excoriated the 'savants' of traditional theory, those who sought to engage in social and political theory without any partisan investment. Resultantly, Critical Theorists, while diagnosing social pathologies, have done so with a consideration of their 'cultural locatedness' and with an explicit awareness of their commitment to political praxis (Bronner, 2011).

Beyond Neuhouser and Honneth, my preferred rebuttal to such challenges would be to return to the approach championed by first generation Critical Theorists, that of immanent-transcendence (Delanty, 2011). While there may be no accord on the good life or what constitutes a functional, or an optimally rational society, through a turn to an immanent-transcendent approach, the theorist may still identify the *objective* contradictions which exist within the social world. With a 'sufficiently dialectical' analysis of said contradictions (Strydom, 2018), in this instance the pathological irrationalities of the social, the theorist can adopt a form of critique which remains sensitive to the disputed nature of social life, while drawing out the objective contradictions of the present, and, through doing so, point towards a more rational future (Chapter Six).

If one accepts the above analyses, the diagnosis of social pathologies, as practised by Critical Theorists, is neither blighted by an unjustifiably strong naturalist ontology, nor destabilised by ethical partisanship. I thus argue that social pathology diagnosing critique offers a social-theoretically and philosophically sound approach to conducting deeper, more foundational social critique beyond the confines of liberal social and political theory.

The Distinctive Utility of Pathology Diagnosing Critique

Diagnosing a social pathology, stating that society is 'sick', and therefore 'irrational' or 'non-functional', is a declaration of something more fundamental than a social injustice. Neuhouser frames this eloquently:

> First, saying that a society is sick involves more than saying that it is unjust. It is not that the category of injustice is always irrelevant to diagnoses of social pathology but rather that, even when considerations of justice are relevant, calling a pathology 'injustice' **under-describes it**. Consider the example of global warming. It would not be unreasonable to regard global warming caused by human activity as an instance of injustice (injustice to future generations, perhaps, or as an injustice on the part of those who profit from the phenomenon to those who merely suffer from it.) It would, however, be a mistake to regard this as an exhaustive description of the problem. This is even more plausible in the case of unsustainably low birth rates, where it is harder to see the problem as one of injustice to future generations since the very problem is that those generations are not going to exist in the first place (Neuhouser, 2012: 629 – my bold).

A diagnosis of social pathology can thus penetrate to core concerns driving social reproduction and submit that something has gone 'gravely awry' with the dominant form of life itself (Neuhouser, 2012: 631). Pathology diagnosing social critique is thus more potent than traditional liberal theory. With the case of global warming, the pathology serves to 'thwart fundamental human end(s)' that are 'deriving from our nature as biological beings' (Neuhouser, 2012: 631). Liberal critiques of injustice crucially lack the purchase, or even the knowledge interest, to engage at this level of analysis. This is perhaps the most intense benefit of adopting a social pathology approach to social critique, it enables the social theorist to ask these deeper, more foundational questions about the social world. Pushing this further, Honneth writes that the diagnoses of social pathology marks 'an instance of reflection … within which measures for successful forms of social life are discussed' (Honneth, 2007c: 4) and, a moment where we focus 'on the appropriateness of our way of life' (Honneth, 2000: 122).

The diagnosis of social pathologies is unique in that it offers Critical Theorists a framework through which both the successfulness and the appropriateness of our ways of life can be assessed, while simultaneously providing a means of engaging with the obstacles to our sound understanding of these problems (Honneth, 2000). To engage with the totality of the social as a system, with its distinct dynamics and modalities, it is essential for the theorist to be able to step back and make such an assessment. The diagnosis of social pathologies is the critical tool that enables such a moment of critical reflection (Honneth, 2000, 2007c).

While Critical Theorists utilise multiple and interlocking disciplines for research, drawing from psychoanalysis, philosophy, social theory, law, politics, geography and psychology, the diagnosis of social pathologies has additional import for Critical Theory as it marks the commonality of the research programme *tout court* (Honneth, 2004). Fromm's psychoanalysis, as much as Fraser's political economy, or Adorno's philosophy, can be grasped, and comprehended, as co-dependent contributions to the project of diagnosing the pathologies of the social. The *Dialectic of Enlightenment,* as much as *The Sane Society,* can thus be held as efforts constructed under a shared horizon. As Honneth (2004a) submits, Critical Theory marks multiple, distinct engagements with the social, that yet all share a foundational basis in the critique of pathologies of the deformed reason of capitalist society.

For Honneth,

> Critical Theorists ... perceive capitalism as a social form of organization in which practices and ways of thinking prevail that prevent the social utilization of a rationality already made possible by history' (Honneth, 2004a: 351).

It is through the diagnosis and analysis of such restrictive processes and modes of thought, that the pathologies of the capitalist form of life can be comprehended. The breadth and profundity of social pathology diagnosis is imperative: as Laitinen submits, pathology diagnosis is essential for a penetrative engagement with the social; the essential fact is 'there is a lot to be criticised in the social reality as it is' (Laitinen, 2015: 48). Critical Theorists require a paradigm which can hold, and enable access to, the totality of the social; to enable the articulation of deformed rationality along the psychoanalytic, political-economic and social theoretical registers.

In this first section, I have argued for the centrality of pathology diagnosing critique throughout the past and present of Critical Theory, and, through a critical exegesis, I have presented the approach as both social-theoretically potent and as philosophically sound.

Recognition Theory: A Focus on the Intersubjective

Having established the significance, and philosophical justifiability, of pathology diagnosing critique, I now engage with the recognition paradigm. In this section I argue that while recognition theory has been of major utility for social theory, it has historically been invoked in to further entirely different concerns to pathology diagnosis. While social pathology diagnosis enables a 'deeper' social critique; recognition theory offers an optic through which to explore the dyadic intersubjective moment, subjectivation and consciousness. I submit that while Honneth's recent radicalisation of the recognition rubric, in *The Struggle for Recognition*, moves to reposition recognition as a way to view the social totality, Honneth's reframing of recognition still does not focus on the core themes of pathology diagnosis. This second section thus outlines what is meant by 'recognition', both prior to, and within, Honneth's framing. This serves to both outline the significance of Honneth's intervention, while marking its continuing distance from the traditional concerns of pathology diagnosing critique.

Consciousness, Subjectivation and Intersubjectivity

Recognition [*Anerkennung*] is perhaps the most debated component of today's socio-theoretical lexicon (Ricoeur, 2005). Indeed, Ricoeur submits that as many as twenty-three different understandings of 'recognition' have been advanced (Ricoeur, 2005: 5-16). Thus, before proceeding further, I present a working definition of recognition for the purposes of this project. For this I turn to Hirvonen (2015), who submits that recognition should be framed as 'positive status attribution that happens *between persons* and (that) also *constitutes* those persons' (Hirvonen, 2015: 210 – original italics). I adopt Hirvonen's accessible construction for it immediately draws out the two components essential to recognition: a) a moment of mutual attribution of positive features between subjects (the intersubjective moment), and b) that this process is essential for subjectivation. This secondary facet, that recognition is 'both responsive to personhood, but at the same time also … constitutes it' (Hirvonen, 2015: 210) informs the ontological commitments of Honneth's Critical Theories of recognition (Ikäheimo, 2007: 227-228). As with my above introduction to social pathology, I offer a brief overview of recognition's role in social theory, drawing out its distinctive concerns: consciousness, intersubjectivity and subjectivation. These are concerns distinct from pathology diagnosing critique, which is identified instead by a desire to conduct 'deeper' social critique.

The orthodox view holds that the 'post-Kantian' imagination of Fichte and Hegel marks the genesis of recognition theorising as practised today (Honneth, 2005; Laitinen, Särkelä and Ikäheimo, 2015: 3). The Fichtean-Hegelian focus of enquiry was the intersubjectively framed moment of subjectivation, and its entwined social-structural realities. In particular, their interest was in how structures of consciousness were socially mediated (Laitinen, Särkelä and Ikäheimo, 2015). As Laitinen, Särkelä and Ikäheimo (2015: 3) draw out, Fichte and Hegel came to hold that, 'through recognition of others, human individuals begin to relate to themselves *and their environment* both epistemically and motivationally' in radically differentiated manners. Recognition became grasped as foundational to the subject's social existence and self-relation. Their enquiry evolved to comprehend society as both product, and creator, of *consciousness*. Hegel and Fichte thus developed conceptual tools to apprehend the patterns and structures of the social as an interconnected whole, and saw recognition, consciousness and subjectivation existing in a proximate relationship.

Hegel is often read as radically expanding Fichte's more 'deontological' understanding of recognition (Laitinen, Särkelä and Ikäheimo, 2015: 4). Most famously, in *The Phenomenology of Spirit*, Hegel introduces a conflictual dimension to the recognition frame: the famous 'struggle for recognition' [*kampf um Anerkennung*] (Hegel 1970: Chapter Four).[13] This much-discussed conflict between 'master' and 'slave', or 'lord' and 'bondsman', centres the themes of dominance and dependency in the recognition register (Kelly, 1966). The subject's foundational, essential recognition is not bestowed with beneficent altruism. Instead, following Hegel, recognition theorists today still point towards an existential 'struggle for recognition'.[14] Drawing upon these Fichtean and Hegelian roots, the idea of recognition, and struggles for its attainment, mark a substantial impact on the Western social-theoretical canon (Kok and van Houdt, 2014).[15] Recognition's reach extends far beyond both left-Hegelian and neo-Hegelian scholarship, and can be seen to have influenced Dewey, Mead and Lacan (amongst others) (Laitinen, Särkelä and Ikäheimo, 2015: 5).

This historical sketch is, inevitably, cursory, and I stress that recognition, just like social pathology diagnosis, carries many layers of complexity (Ikäheimo, 2002; Laegaard, 2005). My submission here is merely that historically, before its rebirth in the latter half of the twentieth century, recognition marked a targeted engagement with the social, focusing on the dyadic intersubjective moment, and the social structural realities connecting consciousness, subjectivation, and the social. While social pathology diagnosis, as discussed, offers a deeper critique of forms of life, through exposing the defective nature of the social totality; recognition theory's philosophical antecedents offer an optic for a more targeted analysis on the relation between subjectivation, consciousness and the intersubjective moment.

From Fichte and Hegel to Taylor and Honneth, recognition offers one point of entry to the social, making no claims nor pretensions to offering a means of engaging with, let alone critiquing, the social totality. To underline this point, Hegel's multifaceted social philosophy, charted in his *Philosophy of Right*, extends far beyond the philosophical and semantic fields of the recognitive (de Boer, 2013).[16] From recognition theory's roots in Fichte and Hegel, one can see the emergence of a body of thought providing an insightful point of entry to the social, through a focus on the intersubjective moment. It is crucial to stress that the philosophical

---

[13] Buck-Morss (2009) suggests that Hegel's framing made have had an antecedent political reality to it, that of the Haitian slave revolts.

[14] Tellingly this is the title of Honneth's central work on the subject.

[15] For example, Chitty (2018) argues that Marx's understanding of 'Species Being' is best understood relative to 'Hegel's view of human beings as conscious subjects who are rationally driven to become universally self-conscious' (Chitty, 2018: 134-135).

[16] De Boer's paper, 'Beyond Recognition? Critical Reflections on Honneth's Reading of Hegel's *Philosophy of Right*' develops this argument with particular relevance to contemporary debates in recognition scholarship.

antecedents to Honneth's recognition theory never presented as an optic to comprehend the social in its totality (Ricouer, 2005). In contrast, this is a claim Honneth repeatedly makes today (Fraser and Honneth, 2001).

While Honneth is the name most associated with contemporary scholarship drawing on recognition (Laitinen, Särkelä and Ikäheimo, 2015: 5-7), it was Charles Taylor's *Multiculturalism and the Politics of Recognition* that brought recognition to the forefront of the contemporary social-theoretical imagination (Heywood, 2007: 316; Martineau, Meer and Thompson, 2012: 2). Through his easy prose, and relatable discussions of new social movements, Taylor reintroduced the recognition paradigm to popular consciousness. To Taylor, recognition is tied intrinsically to identity (Taylor, 1994); the absence of due recognition, 'can inflict harm, can be a form of oppression, imprisoning someone in a false, distorted, and reduced mode of being' (Taylor, 1994: 25). Taylor's essay returned recognition to the centre of social theory, and, with a new, accessible focus on identity, retreated from the Fichtean-Hegelian metaphysics. 'Recognition' offered both social-theorists an efficacious explanatory framing and offered the members of new social movements a rubric for demands, in an intuitive vocabulary. Yet, it must be clarified that for Taylor, recognition did not, and ought not claim to, present as the sole axis for social theoretical analysis or for social action. While the desire for recognition helped frame the claims of the new social movements, Taylor did not present recognition as an optic through which to view the totality of social struggle.

While Taylor returned the recognition framing to the popular imagination, Honneth's *The Struggle for Recognition* is 'generally acknowledged' as 'presenting the most ambitious agenda … utilizing the idea of recognition' in contemporary social theory (Laitinen, Särkelä and Ikäheimo, 2015: 6). Honneth's theory opened the door to a form of social critique which analysed society, *in its entirety*, on the basis of its capacity to enable subjects to achieve the forms of 'primary intersubjective' recognition required for their self-actualisation (Varga and Gallagher, 2012: 243-260). Many scholars go so far as to say that Honneth created an entire Critical Theory derivative the central tenets of the recognition theoretical outlook: a true Critical Theory of Recognition (Alexander and Lara, 1996: 126-136). In the next section, I critically engage with Honneth's contemporary framing of recognition, and argue that, while he radically expands the recognition optic to incorporate the totality of the social, Honneth's approach remains substantially distinct from the pathology diagnosing framing.

From Hegel and Fichte, to Taylor and Honneth, 'recognition', and 'recognition theories' represent an entry point for analysis of the social world through a focus on the intersubjective and its relation to consciousness and identity. This thesis in no way rejects the utility of recognition theory as a point of engagement with identity, consciousness and subjectivation. Instead, following Taylor (1994) and Honneth (2005), I agree that recognition is at the core of the demands of many new social movements, and through a focus on identity, consciousness and subjecthood, recognition centric approaches can provide much needed insight for social-theory. My submission is merely that the knowledge interest of recognition theory, up until Honneth, was limited to a differentiated understanding of consciousness, subjecthood, subjectivation and identity. The philosophical antecedents of Honneth's recognition theory do not offer a paradigm for totalising social critique, a claim which continues to distinguish Honneth's approach, despite its controversiality (Fraser and Honneth, 2001). Simply put, recognition centric analyses offer a distinct engagement with the social, which can be of true utility, but both historically and presently, their concerns are entirely distinct from the diagnosis of social pathologies. As I shall argue, attempts to fuse them have proved damaging to theoretical potency (Chapter Two).

Honneth's Critical Theory of Recognition

Honneth's Critical Theory of recognition was first presented in *Kampf um Anerkennung* (1992) and published in English three years later as *The Struggle for Recognition* (Honneth, 1995). It is worth stressing the work's distinctiveness from both the preceding recognition theoretical approaches and from pathology diagnosing social criticism. *The Struggle for Recognition* marked a radical expansion of recognition theory (Martineau, Meer and Thompson, 2012: 3). Honneth's approach comprehends not only new social movements as recognition struggles, but views all social dynamics, including the explicitly political-economic, through the recognition paradigm (Fraser and Honneth, 2001). I stress that for the early Honneth, 'recognition theory' and 'pathology diagnosis' marked two distinct and evolving endeavours (Freyenhagen, 2015), and thus their dissimilarity, and lack of interpenetration marked no profound anomaly or drawback. In Honneth's earlier work they were simply divergent research interests. It is only when the two come to be elided in the 'pathologies of recognition' approach that problems of such a union for pathology diagnosing critique came to the fore (Chapter Three).[17]

Published seven years before *Kampf um Anerkennung*, Honneth's *Kritik der Macht* argued that the Frankfurt School strain of Critical Theory suffers 'from an exclusive focus on the domain of material production as the locus of transformative critique' (Anderson, 1995: xi). Honneth's long-time translator, Anderson, thus situates *The Struggle for Recognition* as Honneth's

---

[17] As I draw out in Chapter Three, Honneth's interests of 'recognition' and 'social pathology' were fused by other scholars.

'alternative account' (Anderson, 1995: xi), an attempt at transcending, in Martin Jay's words, the Frankfurt School's 'productivist bias' (Jay, 2012: 5). In place of the antecedent materialism, which Honneth saw as ossifying Critical Theory, *Kampf um Anerkennung* moved to centre Critical Theory around 'struggles for recognition' (Anderson, 1995: xi). To this end Honneth radically extends a line of Hegelian thought, part of Hegel's earlier 'Jena writings'. In particular Honneth reanimates *System der Sittlichkeit*; with its distinct recognition centrality (Hegel, 1979). As Anderson's summarises;

> Honneth takes from Hegel the idea that full human flourishing is dependent on the existence of well-established, 'ethical' relations – in particular, relations of love, law, and 'ethical life (*Sittlichkeit*) – which can only be established through a conflict-ridden developmental process, specifically, through a struggle for recognition (Anderson, 1995: xi).

Honneth's key challenge was to build a 'social theory with normative content' derived from these insights of the Jena period Hegel, that would be acceptable in today's 'condition of post-metaphysical thinking' (Honneth, 1995: 1). To do so Honneth drew on Mead's psychology and Winnicott's object-relations theory (Honneth, 1995: 71-91). Utilising empirical psychology, sociology, psycho-analysis and history, Honneth advanced the merits of considering the social as a totality as a network of recognition relations. The legal framework, the market, the systems of familial and erotic love; all now were offered as sites of demands for the intersubjective recognition essential to identity formation and human flourishing. Fundamentally, feelings of 'disrespect' and 'injustice', which catalyse protest and agitation, evince 'relational disorders' that should be 'assessed within the categories of mutual recognition' (Honneth, 1995: 106). Honneth makes this point even more explicit with regards the politico-economic realm in dialogue with Nancy Fraser (Fraser and Honneth, 2001). He states one should 'speak of capitalist society as an institutionalised recognition order' (Fraser and Honneth, 2001: 137); and considers demands for alternative distributions as 'specific kind(s) of struggle for recognition in which the appropriate evaluation of the social contributions of individuals or groups in contested' (Fraser and Honneth, 2001: 171). It seems no exaggeration to state that Honneth's *Struggle for Recognition* marks a radically distinct move in Critical Theory to comprehend all instances of socio-political contestation as instances of 'the expression of a struggles for recognition' (Fraser and Honneth, 2001: 137). Honneth's recognition monism marks a substantial divergence from past recognition framings: Honneth's Critical Theory of Recognition views the totality as the social as a recognition matrix.

In the final chapter of *The Struggle for Recognition* Honneth moves to produce 'A Formal Conception of Ethical Life', dependant on 'the intersubjective conditions' necessary for 'personal integrity' (Honneth, 1995: 171). Yet, the closer Honneth returns to the crucial focus on historically mediated reason, essential to pathology diagnoses, the closer he moves to a paralysing historicism:

> What can count as an intersubjective prerequisite for a successful life becomes historically variable and is determined by the *actual level of development* of the patterns of recognition (Honneth, 1995: 175).

Thus, while the three distinct patterns of recognition (reflecting love, rights and solidarity) represent 'intersubjective conditions that we must further presuppose, if we are to describe the general structures of a successful life' (Honneth, 1995: 175) their realities, and modes, of their granting and apprehension, are products of located historical reality. Yet this reality, and its development is never tied to society as evincing a historically mediated rationality. It is 'the patterns of recognition' which overdetermines social life. In short, Honneth's *Struggle for Recognition* does not provide the tools for social critique which were essential for by previous Critical Theoretical social pathology diagnoses. Recall, pathology diagnosing critique has long been based on a fusion of theoretical frameworks and was consciously practised through a 'multifaceted and polycentric' diagnostic endeavour (Fraser and Honneth, 2001). Honneth's Critical Theory of Recognition does not seek to engage with the totality of the social to diagnose social pathologies. Rather, it seeks to engage solely with 'the development of patterns of recognition' (Honneth, 1995: 175). That this limited, recognition-centric endeavour has come to be conflated with the totality of pathology diagnosing critique is the central theoretical development which this thesis seeks to displace.

It is clear that Honneth's *Struggle for Recognition* marked a radically distinct reorientation of Critical Theory, arguing for a new focus on the essential *ethical* relations necessary for the subject to develop self-confidence, self-respect and self-esteem (Honneth, 1995), it did not offer the tools, or present a desire, to engage in pathology diagnosing critique *qua* Frankfurt School notions of diagnostic critique. In Honneth's recognition theory, the foundational requirements for human flourishing prove to be entirely 'dependent on the establishment of relations of mutual recognition' (Anderson, 1995: xi). Alexander and Lara thus go as far as to frame *The Struggle for Recognition* as a 'philosophical and sociological polemic' (Alexander and Lara, 1996: 127), precisely due to the divergence between Honneth's recognition-centricism and the antecedent frameworks for social critique.

Honneth's *Kampf Um Anerkenung* marked a radical change in the direction of Critical Theoretical scholarship on recognition. Following Honneth, the social totality is now increasingly viewed as a recognition network; and struggles for recognition became a primary means to comprehend not only new social movements, but also the market, and the institutions of the family (Honneth, 1995, 2014b). Yet Honneth's radical extension of the recognition framing did not extend to a direct conflation of recognition theory with the Frankfurt School tradition of pathology diagnosing tradition. *Kampf Um Anerkenung* neither positioned recognition theory as a pathology diagnosing rubric, nor sought to precipitate a synthesis between the two critical theoretical tools. Honneth's analyses, and championing of pathology diagnosis, simply marked a divergent endeavour to his Critical Theory of recognition. While Honneth champions both his radical Critical Theory of recognition, and a reanimation of the pathology diagnosing tradition, it was not his own research that united these framings. That damaging elision, which this thesis critiques, and seeks to displace, was instead performed through a later generation of theorists (Chapter Three).

Conclusion

The chapter has engaged with the central assumptions which undergird the broader project, namely the continuing justifiability and relevance of pathology diagnosing social critique and its natural dissimilarity from recognition theory. Through a cursory outline of the social pathology and recognition-theory traditions, it has demonstrated the richness of these distinct approaches. As this chapter has stressed, Honneth's new Critical Theory of Recognition marks a radical reorientation of the recognition-theoretical framework. It is this new, totalising recognition paradigm that this thesis seeks to critique.

My discussion on the origins of social pathology started with Plato. Perhaps the most famous injunction of the great philosopher was that 'the unexamined life is not worth living' (Plato, 38a5-6). Not only is the desire to conduct a foundational critique of our way of life a central part of being human, but the urgency of this endeavour has never been more pressing. The doomsday clock sits at two minutes to midnight (Mecklin, 2018). Without such foundational reflection, and consonant political practice, the bell risks tolling ever sooner. Society's ability to diagnose its own pathologies is central for the flourishing of social subjects: both because criticism is itself an important form of social existence, but more pressingly, without the ability to diagnose the fundamental social irrationalities, society will continue to be driven by self-destructive, capitalist social logics.

Chapter Two

Honneth's Critical Theory of Recognition: A Critique

Introduction

In this second chapter I critique the recognition-theoretical approach advanced by Honneth (1995, 2014b). By bringing Thompson's (2016) *The Domestication of Critical Theory* into dialogue with existing critiques of recognition theory (Fraser 1995a, 1995b, 2001; McNay 2008, *inter alia*), this chapter argues that exclusively recognition approaches to engaging the social totality are social-theoretically, philosophically, and politically unjustifiable. It is worth reiterating that I do acknowledge the insights offered by alternative recognition approaches. This chapter is not an attempt to invalidate or refute the idea of a 'recognition moment' or the importance of other recognition framings for social theory (past and present). Honneth's approach is distinct from other understandings of recognition in that it is entirely monistic:[18] for Honneth the totality of the social can be grasped through recognition theory. This chapter thus offers a critique targeted at Honneth's *overly-restrictive* recognition approach which excludes alternate approaches to social critique. My thesis proper seeks not the termination of all engagements with recognition. Rather this thesis builds to argue for a 'multilateral' and 'polycentric' Critical Theory which can benefit from a plurality of approaches to engaging with the social, including a modified, non-unifocal recognition lens (Fraser and Honneth, 2001: 209). To restate, the broader aim of this project is to reanimate the Critical Theoretical engagement with social pathologies by displacing the problematically restrictive recognition-derived approach with a more open framing so the full breadth and range of social pathologies can be interrogated. As shall be developed in Chapter Three, the dominant recognition-derived approaches to social pathology diagnosis are predicated upon a restrictive recognition theoretical understanding of the social. The critique of what Fraser terms 'recognition monism' offered in this chapter seeks to destabilise the foundations upon which today's dominant approaches to social pathology are built (Fraser and Honneth, 2001).

As I emphasise throughout this thesis, those[19] who adopt a 'pathologies of recognition' or a recognition-cognitive approach to the social critique 'are convinced that the terms of recognition must represent the unified framework for [the Critical Theoretical] ... project' (Fraser and Honneth, 2001: 113). Drawing heavily on Honneth's Critical Theory of Recognition, they

---

[18] The is the term used repeatedly by Fraser in her debate with Honneth and seems apposite as an adjective considering the unifocal, singular reliance on recognition that Honneth advances (Fraser and Honneth, 2001).
[19] As shall be discussed in Chapter Three, one can see such trends in the 'Jyväskylä School' approach, in the 'Essex School' theorists, and in the recognition-cognitive framing of Zurn (2011).

submit the strong thesis 'that even distributional injustices must be understood as the institutional expression of social disrespect – or, better said, of unjustified relations of recognition' (Fraser and Honneth, 2001: 114). The 'recognition-turn', and the subsequent variegated embrace of such thought, has occurred across traditional disciplinary lines. As a result there have been sparks of resistance within philosophy, gender theory, political theory, psycho-analysis and sociology (McNay, 2008; Fraser and Honneth, 2011; Thompson, 2016). To avoid the limiting effects of arbitrary disciplinary demarcations, I have loosely grouped the critiques of Honnethian recognition approaches into 'political', 'philosophical', and 'social-theoretical' (in contrast to 'gender', 'sociology', 'philosophy', 'psycho-analysis' *inter alia*). I acknowledge the weakness of my typology,[20] and use it apologetically, to provide a clear structure and to unite theoretical concerns which may cross disciplinary boundaries.

This chapter sits in three sections. First, there is a social-theoretical critique of the Honnethian approach to Recognition, second a philosophical critique, third, a critique of the political limitations and contradictions that a unifocal or monistic recognition perspective precipitates. Expressed most simply, this chapter argues that such restrictive recognition approaches are philosophically unjustifiable, limiting to social-theoretical engagement and are politically counter-productive. This chapter is thus essential to my broader thesis as the 'pathologies of recognition' framework, and the ascendant 'recognition-cognitive' approach to social pathology diagnosis (discussed in Chapter Three), are both predicated upon the untenable Honnethian account of recognition.

Social Theoretical Critique

Other distinct structures, other distinct pathologies

For theorists committed to an exclusively recognition account of the social, all societal problems, including distributional irrationalities, 'must be understood as the institutional expression of **social disrespect**', stemming from 'unjustified relations of recognition' (Fraser and Honneth, 2001: 114 – my bold). The entirety of social reality is presented as accessible to the social theorist via the optic of recognition theory (Fraser, 1995a, 1995b; Fraser and Honneth, 2001). Such an approach holds recognition as the 'fundamental overarching' social category and views all other logics and modalities as 'derivative' (Fraser and Honneth, 2001: 2-3). Such recognition accounts seeks 'to subsume the problematic of redistribution (*inter alia*) within' the recognition

---

[20] As stressed in my introduction, Critical Theory has long advocated an interdisciplinary approach. I adopt this subject based division solely for its useful structural demarcations and do so well aware that such an approach has limitations.

theoretical optic (Fraser and Honneth, 2001: 3). All social realities are presented as 'derivate' from fundamental recognition relationships. The role of the social theorist is thus to uncover the 'pathologies of recognition', the instances, and dynamics of 'failures of recognition relationships' and to examine 'the inherent dangers that unstable or ambivalent recognition relationships pose' (Hirvonen, 2015: 209). Drawing on Fraser (1995a, 1995b; Fraser and Honneth, 2001) and McNay (2008), I argue that such an approach fails to account for the existence of the numerous social structures which are not merely epiphenomenal to recognition relationships.[21] Thus, the ascendancy of the pathologies of recognition and recognition-cognitive approaches (Chapter Three), which are predicted on solely recognition-theoretical accounts of the social, seriously impedes the Critical Theoretical diagnosis of social pathologies. If the only social pathologies that are accessible through a solely recognition account are those of the recognition order it undeniably follows that the numerous other species of social pathology: those of political-economy, of consciousness, of the psyche, *inter alia*, are rendered invisible and inaccessible. This thesis submits that it is precisely this elision of important social domains that has served to 'domesticate' pathology diagnosing social critique.

Drawing on Fraser, I directly challenge the Honnethian assertion that all social pathologies must be viewed as stemming from 'unjustified relations of recognition' (Fraser and Honneth, 2001: 114). Following Fraser, while I do not consider economic distribution to be merely epiphenomenal to the recognition order of society; neither do I submit that both social orderings are entirely independent, and hermetically sealed.

> Rather, the economic logic of the market interacts in complex ways with the cultural logic of recognition, sometimes instrumentalising existing status distinctions, sometimes dissolving or circumventing them, and sometimes creating new ones. As a result, market mechanisms give rise to economic class relations that are not mere reflections of status hierarchies (Fraser and Honneth, 2001: 214).

Furthermore,

> Neither those relations nor the mechanisms that generate them can be understood by recognition monism. An adequate approach must theorize both the distinctive dynamics of the capitalist economy and its interaction with the status order (Fraser and Honneth, 2001: 214).

Under scrutiny here is the fundamental legitimacy of the strong thesis advanced by unifocal recognition theorists: that all social inequities and irrationalities can be traced to, and are reflections of, society's antecedent recognition order. In sharp contradistinction, I find Fraser's account entirely more convincing when she submits that 'not all maldistribution is a by-product of misrecognition' (Fraser and Honneth, 2001: 35). To justify this crucial submission Fraser offers the example of a skilled, male, white worker, who becomes unemployed 'due to a factory closing

---

[21] For example, capitalist macro-economic logics.

resulting from a speculative corporate merger' (Fraser and Honneth, 2001: 35).[22] The resultant, potentially mass unemployment that occurs in exactly such situations is best theorised as the result of a multiplicity of factors, including:

> ...the supply and demand for different types of labor [sic]; the balance of power between labor [sic] and capital; the stringency of social regulations, including the minimum wage; the availability and cost of productivity enhancing technologies; the ease with which firms can shift their operations to locations where wage rates are lower; the cost of credit; the terms of trade; and international currency exchange rates (Fraser and Honneth, 2001: 215).

Following Fraser, I submit that viewing this plethora of political-economic factors (not to mention the complex constellation of non-political economic factors, many of which are equally distanced from the recognition order) as expressions of the recognition order, is unjustifiable. Rather, these political-economic factors are best theorised as a result of logics inherent to the dominant form of capitalist economy (Thompson, 2016). In such cases it seems incontrovertible that deeply significant social actions occur with momentous material repercussions that have 'little to do with recognition' (Fraser and Honneth, 2001: 35). The importance of the operation of such capitalist logics, which are at the very least once-removed from the status order, cannot be underplayed. As Fraser suggests, the 'distinguishing feature' of capitalist modernity is the 'creation of a quasi-autonomous, impersonal market order that follows a logic of its own' (Fraser and Honneth, 2001: 24): a logic which is not merely epiphenomenal to the given society's recognition order. This is not to claim, or to underprivilege, the significance of status, identity, or recognition to social reproduction, or to underinvest in the academic utility of their study and analysis. Rather, my submission is that the dominant trend to focus *solely* on 'pathologies of recognition' restricts the capacity of the social theorist to engage with, and expose, the numerous genera of social pathologies that exist in the various other social-structures which operate contemporaneously and non-epiphenomenally, to the recognition order.

As first and second-generation Critical Theorists submitted, there are pathologies of the political-economic order itself (Held, 1980; Strydom, 2011). The grand thesis of *Capital* may even be read as Marx's prediction that the capitalist system would fall under the weight of its own pathologies (Honneth, 2007c). Such 'social pathologies of the economy' may include *inter alia* self-perpetuating dynamics of negative infinity, a trend towards overall immiseration, or the systemic reward of consumption irrespective of the cost to other social goods (Neuhouser, 2012). It is evident that such pathologies are not accessible through a solely recognition

---

[22] Fraser's hypothetical worker is white, male and working in an esteemed job, to represent an ideal-typical individual who does not suffer from 'misrecognition'.

register,[23] for they are not 'pathologies of recognition'. Rather they are pathologies fundamental to the economic order, which exist non-epiphenomenally to the recognition order.

As subsequent chapters of this thesis will advance, the dominant recognition-derived approach to social pathology diagnosis, and to social theory more broadly, obscures a plethora of important social dynamics (Chapters Four to Six). Chapter Four explores Rousseau's foundational social theory, drawing out the existence of multiple framings of social pathology which are entirely inaccessible to recognition-centric approaches. Perhaps the most obvious candidate for social-theoretical scholarship which is invisible to the recognition-monist approach is the presence of (non-recognitive) social-structural dynamics. Neuhouser (2012) locates such a species of social pathology in Rousseau's *Discourse of Political Economy*, exemplified below:

> ... in order to raise ... armies, tillers had to be taken off the land; the shortage of them lowered the quality of the produce, and the armies' upkeep introduced taxes that raised its price. This first disorder caused the people to grumble: in order to repress them, the number of troops had be increased and, in turn, the more despair increased, the greater the need to increase it still more in order to avoid its consequences (c.f. Neuhouser, 2012: 11).

Here we have a species of social pathology, a self-perpetuating negative dynamic, that is not observable through recognition accounts, and one which has little, if anything, to do with the recognition register. Both farmers and soldiers may be esteemed and recognised, and nothing would change, for the pathology exists in a deeper social dynamic, not at an intersubjective register. As left-Hegelians would argue, the problem is simply an irrationality in social organisation (Chapter Five). Further pathological dynamics invisible to the recognition approach are engaged with by Fromm (Chapter Six). Fromm's account of 'pathological normalcy' is important in that it combines a Marxian critique of the irrationalities and limitations in the objective social order with the pathologies of the ideological realm which lead to the societal dynamics of normalisation and quiescence (Fromm, 1963). Consider, for instance, Stanley Kubrick's dark satirical comedy, written contemporaneously to Fromm's *The Sane Society, Dr. Stranglelove or: How I learned to Stop Worrying and Love the Bomb*. In the denouement, when the war committee is discussing an impending nuclear apocalypse and the need to restart civilisation in protected underground bunkers, an interesting dialogue occurs, indicative of this subset of social pathologies which exists entirely beyond the recognition register. General 'Buck' Turgidson (George C. Scott) and Dr. Strangelove (Peter Sellers) discuss the need to prevent a 'mineshaft gap'.[24] This is, of course, a dark satirical extension of 'the arms race'. For Fromm, this

---

[23] Interestingly, a recent paper claims to frame similar logics through exactly such a recognition lens (Schaub and Odigbo, 2019). I critique the manifold failings of this attempt in Chapter Three.
[24] The joke here is that while for decades the Soviet Union and the United States had been racing to stockpile more and more nuclear weapons, in a dynamics which had developed beyond the control of either superpower, a similar

dialogue would be seen as depicting two species of pathology, neither accessible to a solely recognition account. Instead, we have a psychological pathology (that such a dynamic is accepted as a norm) and secondly, and a species of pathology in social functioning more broadly. The 'mineshaft gap', as with the 'nuclear gap' represents a species of damaging negative dynamic, which, annexed to the socially imbued and perpetuated pathological paranoia, risks becoming a dynamic of negative infinity.

These examples are merely indicative of the breadth and depth of framings of social pathology which are obscured by the Honnethian recognition approach to social critique. As expressed throughout subsequent chapters on Rousseau (Chapter Four), Hegel (Chapter Five) and Fromm (Chapter Six) the full *genera* of social pathologies is perhaps limitless, and the artificial restraints of the Honnethian recognition imaginary must urgently be challenged and repudiated to regain social-theoretical potency. The contemporary dominance of the recognition approach to social-theory restricts access to crucial aspects of social reality, leading to a 'telescoped' Critical Theory (Thompson, 2016: 6). Restrictive Critical Theories of Recognition are thus social-theoretically unsound as they fail to account for the multiplicity of distinct social processes and modalities which are not merely epiphenomenal to the recognition order. This is a social-theoretical weakness which is unsurmountable which lies at the heart of Honneth's approach.

On the dangerous allure of unifocal social theory

Part of the problem with restrictive recognition accounts may stem from the desire to find a unitary category of analysis to start with. Drawing on Fraser, I submit there are reasonable grounds to 'object in principle to *any* proposal to ground a normative framework on one privileged set of experiences' (Fraser and Honneth, 2001: 205 – original italics). A social theory which commits to a singular optic for understanding social reality 'puts all its eggs in one basket' (Fraser and Honneth, 2001: 205) from the start. Once a commitment has been made to an approach, the temptation is thus to stretch it, to attempt to incorporate too much within its confines. This is precisely what Critical Theories of recognition have been accused of: 'inflat(-ing) the idea of recognition to the point of unrecognizability (sic), thereby draining it of critical force' (Fraser and Honneth, 2001: 210; Thompson, 2016).

---

dynamic could occur where each power sought to hold the most underground sites for survival (mineshafts were considered a potentially safe place to be during a nuclear conflict).

While this is perhaps excessively generalising, broad-brush analysis, there are undeniable advantages to supporting a 'polycentric and multilateral' Critical Theory (Fraser and Honneth, 2001: 209), the approach this thesis champions. There is no need to push for a singular optic, it provides no greater insight compared to polycentric approaches to the social. Unicentric recognition accounts which purport the primacy of an '*a priori monism*' of recognition serve to artificially restrict social theoretical engagement (Fraser and Honneth, 2001: 210). A strong critique of monistic approaches to the social is that they privilege a singular entry point to social reality, necessarily offering a singular set of parameters for comprehension. When, inevitably, the contingent messiness of social reality is too complex for a singular framework, theorists committed to the strategy redefine terms, and stretch parameters, leaving their original insight distorted beyond recognition (McNay, 2008: 195). Such a critique of restrictive recognition accounts is entirely justified, for they 'illegitimately' serve to 'totalize one mode of integration, truncating the full range of social process', and thus obscures the full spectrum and genera of social dynamics and their attendant pathologies (Fraser and Honneth, 2001: 214).

McNay goes as far as to submit that recognition theorists have fallen victim to what Bourdieu termed 'scholastic epistemo-centricism' (Bourdieu 2000: 52; McNay 2008: 195). This is a general tendency which can occur in social theory where theorists develop such an investment in an approach that the 'specificity of social practice is neutralized' so as to enable it to be 'assimilated to an intellectual construct' (McNay, 2008: 195). Not only can a critique be offered to the claim that the struggle for recognition is a constant 'archetype whose fundamental dynamic is superimposed on all … social relations' but the very nature of the dynamic shifts arbitrarily as desired (McNay, 2008: 51). It becomes increasingly unclear what 'recognition' means as it needs to be constantly redefined, sometimes 'beyond all recognition' (Ricoeur, 2005: 5-16).

The complexity of social reality cannot be grasped by a singularly recognitive account, because no unifocal approach to conducting social theory can access the totality of the social. All theoretical approaches come with their attendant limitations. Many in the current generation of recognition theorists, in their desire to comprehend the breadth of social reality within their singular recognition framework do damage to their very conception of social reality to stay 'true' to their approach. In this regard restrictive recognition approaches to the social epitomise 'scholastic epistemocentricism' (McNay, 2008: 195).

Restrictive recognition accounts are social-theoretically unjustifiable in that they fail to access the range of social processes and structures that constitute social reality. Through these omissions, the precipitant recognition-derived engagements with social pathology occlude the economic, psycho-analytic and social logics which occur beyond the recognition order. McNay

(2008) suggests that recognition theorists' devotion to their framing despite these obvious failings can be explained through reference to the tendency to 'scholastic epsitemocentricism'. Restrictive recognition-derived engagements with the social world thus do damage to their own comprehension of social reality in order to stay 'true' to their desired approach.

Philosophical Critique

Having advanced a social-theoretical critique of the dominant recognition theoretical approach to social theory, the chapter now presents a philosophical critique. To reiterate, the division of this chapter into social-theoretical, philosophical, and political is admittedly imperfect, and at best crudely functional. While the social-theoretical section focused on the critiques of the unifocal recognition framing as an inadequate means of theorising society, my philosophical critique focuses on the neo-Idealist assumptions and ontological claims that the unifocal recognition approach necessitates.

Uniting Thompson (2016), McNay (2008), and Fraser (1995a, 1995b, 2001) this section argues that restrictive Critical Theories of recognition are predicated upon damagingly 'reductive understanding(s) of power' (McNay, 2008: 2). The Honnethian recognition approach unjustifiably distances human sociality from 'concrete social structures and mechanisms' (Thompson, 2016: 5). Honneth's approach is found wanting because recognition does not occur in a vacuum, hermetically sealed from market forces. The diagnosed 'pathologies of recognition' which follow from such an account, those (relative few) which are even observable within said optic, are thus philosophically limited: they are predicated on illegitimately extracting the recognition dyad from broader, non-recognition based, social processes. Utilising Thompson's critique of 'neo-Idealism' (Thompson, 2016, 2019), I argue that the monistic recognition account necessitates indefensible ontological commitments and precipitates an 'ahistorical' and 'reductive' understanding of subject formation (McNay, 2008: 24). My primary submission is that recognition monists, those who express the causal, ontological and moral primacy of the intersubjective dyad, necessarily disconnect social pathologies 'from a socio-structural account of power' (McNay, 2008: 9). Further, drawing on McNay (2008), Connell (1987) and Fraser (1995a, 1995b, 2001), I argue that recognition monists present a false universal commonality to social existence, submitting that an identical intersubjective dynamic can be located cross-culturally. Such an understanding is *prima facie* rejected in light of historical and social contingency, and the complexities of non-standard human subjects, for example: infants, the enslaved, or those with serious learning difficulties. Finally, I submit that recognition theoreticians' claims that the optic of recognition solves the 'theory-immanent problem'

(Honneth, 2001: 125-6) is unjustifiable. I end my philosophical critique of Honneth's recognition monism by submitting there exists no immanent 'body of pristine experience in inchoate everyday suffering' with which social theorists can align progressive scholarship (Fraser and Honneth, 2001: 203). The imperatives of systems and structures that 'pulse beneath the surface of everyday life' (Thompson, 2016: 7) are coeval with human sociality, shaping consciousness, subjectivation and intersubjectivity. Fundamentally, the Honnethian recognition account is crippled by its ontological commitment to the primacy of the dyadic recognition moment: such an approach is a wilful negation of the constant impact of power, especially systemic-structural imperatives, on all facets of human existence.

Neo-Idealism and the ontological commitments of Honnethian recognition theory

As established in Chapter One, Honnethian recognition theorists, in keeping with Third Generation Critical Theory more broadly, seek a 'pure kernel' of social existence from which to enter the social conjecture (Thompson, 2016). For recognition monists this point of entry is the intersubjective moment of recognition. Honneth, for instance, is explicit in the causal, ontological and moral primacy he accords the 'moment' of intersubjective praxis (Honneth, 1995, 2014). He posits a fundamental, 'primal dyad', which 'lies at the at the origin of social relations' (McNay, 2008: 47). The recognition of subject A by subject B, and, simultaneously, of subject B by subject A, is held to be the optimum point of entry to social reality for critical scholarship as it marks the genesis of social being (Honneth, 1995; McNay, 2008).

These is a clear ontological claim here: for recognition theorists, society is held to be nothing more than 'extrapolations of psychic dynamics' (McNay, 2008: 138). Society is determined by, and is best conceived as, a 'recognition order' (Honneth, 1995, 2014). The importance placed on the intersubjective dyad is staggering: recognition marks nothing less than the originary point of the social[25] *and*, for Honneth, it is the entirety of the social. For recognition theorists, there is a 'unidirectional causal dynamic' to the 'ontology of recognition' (McNay, 2008: 138): everything flows outward from the recognition moment. Thus, the intersubjective relations of recognition between subjects instigates, comprises, determines and perpetuates the dominant form of social reality. For recognition monists the primal dyadic relationship comes first in all aspects of social philosophy: it is recognition relationships that constitute subjectivities and human sociality. From such a viewpoint it logically follows for the site of analysis, and thus of social critique, to shift to the cognitive and noumenal capacities essential for intersubjective praxis.

---

[25] Recall how all foundational subjectivation requires a recognition relationship.

Thus, with the Third Generation of Critical Theory there is a new-found (and mis-placed) faith in the emancipatory and critical powers of the cognitive and the intersubjective (Thompson, 2016).

In *The Domestication of Critical Theory* (2016) Thompson critiques this movement of the primary site of Critical Theoretical analysis as evincing a 'neo-Idealist' social ontology (Thompson, 2016).[26] Thompson defines 'neo-Idealism' as,

> ... (a school of thought where) ... thinkers proceed from the premise that *there is a self-sufficiency* to the powers of intersubjective reason, discourse, structures of justification, and recognition (Thompson, 2016: 15 – my italics).

In addition to the word 'self-sufficiency', one could add the adjectives 'potency' and 'purity'. At core here is that neo-Idealists invest the cognitive realm with an ability to avoid penetration by the 'potency of social power, rooted in the material organization of social life' (Thompson, 2016: 15). They contend that the strictures of social structure do not impede the cognitive domain, nor in any way corrupt or tarnish its emancipatory potential. The intersubjective moment is held to be simply infallible. It is with this belief they fall into, what Thompson describes as, the 'neo-idealist fallacy'. Contemporary recognition theorists invest 'modern subjects with powers of rationality ... (they) *simply cannot possess*' (Thompson, 2016: 5 – my italics). 'The crucial flaw' of such neo-Idealist thought,

> is that it detaches itself from a theory of socialization that is actually fused to the concrete structures of social power and its capacity to shape consciousness and cognition (Thompson, 2016: 3).

For neo-Idealists, certain facets of subjectivity, and sociality, are not shaped and determined by social structures, and can thus be invested with radical emancipatory potential. This is based on an unjustifiable social ontology: social being is not solely derived from recognition relationships. The cognitive capacities of subjects are created and shaped by broader social-structural logics (Thompson, 2016: 3-5). In light of Thompson's critique, it seems evident that Honnethian recognition theory is predicated upon an unsustainable social ontology and a theory of subjectivation which is congenitally blind to the impact of power, particularly 'constitutive power', upon subjects.

This return to the cognitive, as recognition monists advance, fundamentally negates the foremost philosophical insight of Marxian philosophy. Recognition monists fail to account for Marx's materialist inversion of Hegelian Idealism, that:

> It is not the consciousness of men that determines their existence, but their social existence that determines their consciousness (Marx, 2010 (1859): 92).

---

[26] The critique is levelled at 'contemporary critical theory' (broadly synonymous with Third Generation Critical Theory), however in a latter article Thompson focuses explicitly on the neo-Idealism in Critical Theories of recognition (Thompson, 2017).

Ever since Marx's Copernican insight it has been apparent that the cognitive facets essential to intersubjective recognition are determined by subjects' material worlds. There is no pristine cognitive capacity which is excluded from the corrupting effects of social systems. In Thompson's words, neo-Idealists fail to engage with how 'concrete social structures ... exert formative pressure on socialization and consciousness' (Thompson, 2016: 5). I contend that the 'pathologies of recognition' that are produced by the Honnethian recognition account are philosophically untenable and fail to engage with the reality that social structures are not merely epiphenomenal to a foundational recognition dyad. In accord with Thompson, Bollenbeck (2019) thus argues that Honneth's Theory of Recognition serves to turn Hegel on its head 'and back again', returning Critical Theory to pure Hegelian Idealism.

Honnethian recognition accounts are thus philosophically unjustified in that they cast the intersubjective moment as untouched by the power emanating from systemic-structural processes. In short, this chapter argues that a social ontology is required that comprehends society as more than just the extension of primal intersubjective dynamics. The constant presence of structural-systemic logics, coeval with subjectivation, will forever frustrate restrictive, unifocal recognition theorists, who hunt the untouched 'intersubjective moment'. The implicit ontological commitments of Honnethian recognition theorists, to viewing society as nothing more than extensions of the primal recognition dyad, which itself remain always pure and untouched,[27] is destabilised once one embraces the Marxist insight of the impact of social structure on consciousness. Honnethian recognition theorists appeal to a fictive 'kind of subjectivity that has not been shaped and formed by defective social relations and institutions' (Thompson, 2016: 6). Such an understanding fails to account for the complex reality of power, and the way in which subjectivities are constituted, coeval with power, rather than independent to, and isolated from, power. This understanding is based on an unjustifiable social ontology, which echoes back to Hegelian Idealism as clearly as Honneth himself returns to Hegel's Jena writings. Thompson's *Domestication of Critical Theory* is an essential intervention in that it reintroduces the two centuries of scholarship since Hegel, reminding Critical Theorists of the essential Marxist insight that 'power relations rooted in capitalist forms of economic life structure the deeper socialization processes that shape the cognitive dimension of the personality of subjects' (Thompson, 2016: 64).

The social ontology and precipitant theory of subjectivation the Honnethian paradigm necessitates is philosophically unjustifiable as it falls into a brazen neo-Idealism. That Critical

---

[27] This problematic investment in a flawless area of the social can be seen to recur with Honneth's (2014) framing of 'social freedom' in *Freedom's Right*.

Theorists have been so keen to obviate the essential hallmark of Marxist scholarship, the importance of the social world on consciousness, seems terrifying. In this regard McNay frames the problem of the dominant recognition approaches beautifully when she argues that it casts 'power relations ... [as] a post hoc effect' (McNay, 2008: 47) on consciousness. McNay continues,

> the ontology of recognition understands the sources of inequality as generated through an interpersonal dynamic of struggle, but this face to face dynamic is disconnected from a socio-structural account of power (McNay, 2008: 47-48).

It is simply untenable to cast power as 'an exogenous factor that come to operate *post hoc* upon the recognition dynamic' instead of being held as fundamentally 'intrinsic' to all social life (McNay, 2008: 72)

Universal Primal Dyad

Recognition monists contend that there is an essential ontological antecedent to *all* human sociality: all 'social relations are seen as extrapolations from primal psychic dynamics' (McNay, 2008: 19). A recognises B, who simultaneously recognises A, and from the continuing expansion of such recognition relationships social relations, and society, is created. The struggle for recognition is presented as both universal and constant. This ultimately (if successful) symmetrical primal relationship is submitted as a fundamental, human, anthropological fact. Drawing on McNay (2008), Fraser (Fraser and Honneth, 2001), Connell (1987) and Fanon (1952), I argue that this presentation presents a false universal commonality to social existence. In light of historical contingency, and the complexities of the myriad subject positions which problematise the posited symmetrical 'primal dyad', I argue that Honnethian recognition theorists offer an ahistorical understanding of the social, blind to socio-cultural variation (Fraser and Honneth, 2001). Connell (1987), for instance, strongly argues that there is tremendous variation to the patterns and logics of oppressive social structures. Even if one were to accede that the antecedent core to all social action was a primary recognition dyad, a strong thesis which requires substantial, as yet unprovided, justification (which I have rejected above); this dyadic relationship would surely be mediated, and susceptible to socio-cultural variation. The idea that at core, all social relations can be reduced to a primal psychic dyadic relationship, which is constant in formation, and equally necessary for the attainment of an anthropological need across cultures, seems philosophically untenable in light of socio-cultural difference.

Fanon's analysis of the psycho-analytic dimension of colonial oppression in *Black Skin, White Masks*, helps illustrate the problems of entrenching the 'primacy of recognition anthropologically, below the level of historical contingency' (Fraser and Honneth, 2001: 206,

McNay, 2008).[28] Extending McNay, I read Fanon as arguing that there can never be a moment of Hegelian recognition in the colonial context, between coloniser and colonial subject. The potential to attain subjecthood through intersubjective praxis is never presented, for there is never the possibility of a moment of mutuality. In McNay's reading, the 'overwhelming power inequalities [in coloniality] annihilate' the possibility of recognition (McNay, 2008: 55); therefore 'it is not the struggle for recognition that forms the subjectivity of the colonial subject but social subordination' (McNay, 2008: 55). The 'crushing object-hood' of 'blackness' locks the colonial subject into oppressive psychic dynamics; there is no potential for transcendence or emancipation through intersubjective praxis (Fanon, 1952: 60). The fundamental dyadic relationship is unattainable in the contingent life-world of the colonial subject. But, *pace* the (implicit) convictions of Honnethian recognition theorists, the absence of the possibility of such relations does not preclude radical, agentival subjectivites, capable of myriad acts of resistance (Fanon, 1952). The struggle simply is 'not personal but social' (Fanon, 1952: 215, c.f. McNay, 2008: 55). For Fraser, such examples are proof that the unifocal recognition theorists assertion that 'one single motivation [recognition]' underlies social action is *prima facie* untenable (Fraser and Honneth, 2001: 203). The example of the contingent impossibility of recognition within the colonial context, yet, simultaneously the very real capacity for struggle and for radical subjectivity, poses a challenge to Honneth (Coulthard, 2014). In this example there are subjects existing in a reality where the impossibility of mutuality precludes the possibility of a moment of intersubjective praxis. That the form of sociality occurring in such a situation is an extension of primal dyadic relations of recognition seems implausible and characterising such a conjecture as subjects 'struggling for recognition' negates the phenomenological and structural realities of the contingent moment. To claim such realities remain epiphenomenal to primal dyadic relations of recognition, or struggles thereof, seems both 'a-historical' and 'reductive' (McNay, 2008: 24).

One further complication for those claiming the universality and primacy of the dyadic relationship posited by recognition monists is that it is unclear that all subjects attain the 'level of consciousness that the model seems to require' (McNay: 2008: 134). The relationship between mother and child, essential to the recognition theoretical psychoanalytic theory of Jessica Benjamin, for example, necessitates cognitive capacities in the infant which cannot be empirically ascertained. Further, there exist countless mature subjects, with rich socialities, that

---

[28] Theorists have also utilised Fanon to critique how recognition politics plays out in particular locations. For instance, Coulthard's (2014) *Red Skin, White Masks* draws upon Fanon to critique the recognition paradigm through a targeted engagement with how recognition-derived political engagements have harmed the indigenous Canadian population.

have cognitive impairments (consider those with severe learning difficulties or disabilities). One cannot commit to the claim that these subjects possess the cognitive capacities essential to intersubjective praxis. It is thus philosophically questionable, as well as politically problematic, to necessitate the degree of consciousness needed for intersubjective praxis as a precondition for entry into the social community.

The argument here, juxtaposing and extending McNay, Fraser, Connell and Fanon, is that the commonality recognition theorists attribute to all social existence is philosophically problematic. Blind to socio-cultural variation, and the social existences of subjects with limited cognitive capacities, recognition monists attributes a false commonality to social existence, which further impedes the optic's philosophical legitimacy.

An Immanent Entry Point for Social Critique?

My final philosophical critique of the Honnethian recognition approach is to challenge its claim to be a 'solution' to the 'theory-immanent problem' (Fraser and Honneth, 2001: 125-6). For Celikates (2018), Critical Theory remains trapped by an unhelpful methodological dichotomy. There are two dominant approaches to social critique.[29] There is 'external' or 'transcendent' critique, which situates itself beyond 'ideology', viewing the everyday social actors as 'judgemental dupes' (Celikates, 2018). Such an approach is typified by Bourdieu's critical sociology, which seeks to diagnose false consciousness and societal maladies from beyond the immediate frame of reference of the social world through academic abstraction. Alternatively, there is the 'internal' or 'immanent' approach which 'follows the actors': such an approach is typified by Garfinkels' ethnomethodology and Boltanski's sociology of critique (Celikates, 2018: 95). As Celikates (2018) outlines, both approaches have their limitations.[30]

For Honneth, the Critical Theory of Recognition is the solution. Recall that for Honneth a clear 'moral injustice is at hand whenever, contra to their expectations, human subjects are denied the recognition they feel they deserve' (Honneth, 2007a: 71). In these feelings of intersubjective disrespect, for recognition monists, one can access the 'moral grammar' of human sociality (Honneth, 1995). For Honneth, focusing Critical Theoretical scholarship on X's feelings of misrecognition, enables social theory to be tied both more closely to the immanent 'normative objectives of emancipatory movements' (Fraser and Honneth, 2001: 113) while retaining an objectivity through the focus on the 'moral grammar' of recognition. In the eyes of recognition

---

[29] Beyond immanent-transcendence which is the methodology championed by Critical Theory (Strydom, 2011).
[30] For my critique of Celikates' proposed solution, see Harris (2019).

theorists, by tracing the claims of denied intersubjective recognition, articulated by such movements, the theorist can locate an immanent entry point for their social critique. If this claim was justifiable it would prove a real strength of recognition theory and would represent a truly meritorious advance in critical social theory. The 'pathologies of recognition' diagnosed by recognition monists would thus carry the extra legitimacy of a direct connection to the immanent claims of the life-world, and, simultaneously, track the quasi-objective, anthropologically legitimated, 'moral grammar' of recognition.

In contrast, I argue that such claims are entirely specious, and that, contrary to such repeated claims to immanence, recognition monism 'serves more' to legitimate a 'metaphorical hall of mirrors for the self', where 'selves that are pathologically shaped by/through culture' are deemed aspirational and legitimate (Thompson, 2016: 65). Opposing recognition-theoretical approaches, I argue both the immanent, the transcendent and the immanent-transcendent approaches are vastly superior methodologies to conducting social critique. Returning once again to Thompson's critique of neo-Idealism, I argue that recognition monists fail to provide the immanent basis to social criticism that they proclaim, for they fail to grasp the true impact of social systemic power on consciousness and cognitive capacities. Yet again, the neo-idealist nature of recognition theory is responsible for the failure of another of its claimed benefits.

What complicates Honneth's claim is that it is instantly apparent that there exists both 'justified and unjustified claims for recognition' (Fraser and Honneth, 2001: 27). For example, justified claims may include the demands for recognition from those fighting racial, sexist, or homophobic abuse. Consider the case of black worker X, subjected to dehumanising, racist abuse in her working environment. X's claim for recognition seems immediately justifiable. In such a scenario the recognition monist's claim to have discovered an immanent entry point for social critique seems entirely justified: demands for recognition seemingly provide an excellent point of entry for critiquing social reality. Yet, then consider the case of the racist, white supervisor, Y, who feels 'disrespected' and 'unrecognised' due to his black staff looking him in the eye, and thus refusing to act in a manner respectful to his self-perceived 'innate superiority'. Both subjects may experience similar emotions of humiliation, may feel disrespected, and feel they have a justified claim that the existing recognition order fails them. Recognition monism fails to provide an immanent point of entry to the social, for it fails to provide any clear determining logic as to which immanent claims are legitimate. There is no neat textbook of objective 'moral grammar' one can consult. On the contrary, such a judgement is made transcendent to the life-world, entirely 'above', or 'outside' the immanent social realm. The Critical Theory of Recognition thus slides back into transcendent critique.

The knowledge that both subjects feel disrespected is thus of limited utility to the social theorist. Indeed, investing either subject X's, or subject Y's sentiment with undue critical potency risks 'simply reproducing the basic validity of the social reality that already exists' (Thompson, 2016: 25). One must ask where each of their feelings of disrespect originate from. Both subject X and subject Y have been socialised into a society fundamentally shaped by 'structural and functional power relations that are routinized (sic) by the prerogatives and goals of social systems' (Thompson, 2016: 66). For Thompson (2016) subjects' feelings of disrespect reflect the dominant sentiments and value-horizons that have been inculcated in their contingent, ideologically buttressed social order. McNay extends Bourdieu to advance a similar critique (McNay, 2008). For Bourdieu, 'the most personal is the most impersonal' (1992: 201): the degree to which subject X's passion is inflamed by occurrence Y, the more clearly the social theorist can witness the primacy of Y to the broader social order. McNay extends Bourdieu's notion of 'habitus': the idea that there are culturally imbibed dispositions, tastes, preferences, and values, which are related to various cultural and class logics, to demonstrate the extent to which what one finds 'insulting' or 'disrespectful' is entirely culturally mediated. From such a perspective, what one finds erotic, distasteful, repulsive, or 'disrespectful' reflects cultural norms and is intrinsically linked to social structures. There is thus no 'prelapsarian knowledge', no 'pure', 'true', definite, immanent life-world oppression that social theory can effortlessly track courtesy of the insights of recognition theory (Berlant, 2000: 43, McNay, 2008: 141).

Without some mediating methodological commitment to ascertain critical value, subjects' feelings of 'disrespect', and 'misrecognition' fail to offer a direct entry point to social reality, rather, to the contrary, they merely throw up the true contingent, ideology-ridden, messiness of the social realm (Celikates, 2018). While both the immanent and the transcendent approaches are aware of this problematic, the Honnethian inspired approach is paralysed in that it fails to acknowledge that it too suffers from the theory-immanent problem. Ultimately Honneth's theory, when applied to the social world, relies upon transcendent moral judgements,[31] eventually an ideologically interpellated human makes a call that 'this recognition claim is (in)valid', that it does or does not track the moral grammar.[32]

McNay and Thompson, despite disciplinary distinctions, produce very similar argumentation: theorists always search in vain if they seek some 'pure', unmediated 'prelapsarian' moral grammar which is objectively being 'disrespected'. Embodied subjectivites feel disrespect due

---

[31] This is also the weakness of Celikates' proposed critique as social practice.
[32] I return to this point in Chapter Seven, where I argue that this fundamental weakness of recognition theory could be utilised as a strength, if the entire recognition approach was inverted.

to the social valuations placed on various behaviour patterns. To determine which feelings of 'disrespect' are to be social-theoretically supported requires complex social-theoretical analysis, which is at best one order removed from the direct claims of immanent politico-social groups. Ultimately Thompson's critique of the neo-Idealism inherent to Honneth's approach invalidates almost all of the purported strengths of the recognition theoretical approach.

Political Critique

Framing social movements as campaigns for liberation from 'pathologies of recognition' has political, as well as philosophical and social-theoretical, weaknesses (Fraser, 1995a, 1995b; Coulthard, 2014; Thompson, 2016). First, I argue that the move to a solely recognition approach represents both a symbolic and a real retreat from the critique of political economy. Even if the system mechanics of neoliberalism could be incorporated within recognition monism, as Honneth contends (Fraser and Honneth, 2001), it would still be framed as epiphenomenal to, rather than fundamental to, the core logics of social reproduction. Second, I argue the species of 'recognition politics' that contemporary recognition approaches are allied to, risks pitting progressive political causes unnecessarily at odds. Drawing on the Fraser-Young debate, I submit that the 'affirmative-transformative' contradiction has validity, although Fraser's (incidental) examples may be counterproductive. The argument forwarded here is that the Honnethian recognition approach, and the recognition-derived approaches it precipitate, are politically problematic and counterproductive.

A retreat from the Critique of Political Economy

First-generation Critical Theorists sought to 'explode the reified forms of thought' (Thompson, 2016: 10) engendered by the capitalist mode of production, and, by doing so, to contribute towards the transition to a more rational social organisation. In such an effort they sought an excoriating critique of the 'organised forms of power that reproduce social pathologies' (Thompson, 2016: 3). When one reads the texts of the first generation of Critical Theorists, Thompson's phrase 'organised forms of power', can be read as largely synonymous with 'market society'. The early Critical Theoretical project was at core political, representing a direct challenge to both the logics of capitalist economic relations and to those who supported them. With a unique fusion of theory and praxis, and with a hyperawareness of their location within ideology; early Critical Theorists saw the very process of articulating the pathological state of consciousness as an essential praxis: as an oppositional act to capitalist domination. Lukacs'

History and Class Consciousness, is but one example amongst many which explicitly ties the project of articulating the pathologies of the social to an assault on the structures of capitalist political economy. As Lukacs expresses at the start of 'Reification and the Consciousness of the Proletariat':

> Our intention here is to *base* ourselves on Marx's economic analyses and to proceed from there to a discussion of the problems growing out of the fetish character of commodities, both as an objective form and also as a subjective stance corresponding to it. **Only by understanding this can we obtain a clear insight into the ideological problems of capitalism and its downfall** (Lukacs, 1972: 84 – original italics, my bold).

The hostility to the capitalism could hardly be expressed any clearer. The 'confrontation with the forms of organized power that reproduce social pathologies', as expressed by Thompson, is instantly visible (Thompson, 2016: 3).

The critique of political economy that was central to classical Critical Theory does not have the same resonance for today's recognition theorists. This is not merely incidental: I contend that not only has the critique of capitalism been largely decentred, but, further, with the ascendancy of a restrictive recognition approach, the very attitude to capitalism has shifted. Honneth even speaks of capitalism as possessing emancipatory potential through the recognition relationships furthered by the market itself (Honneth, 2014b: 208; Conclusion). My argument here is that the 'domestication' of Critical Theory's politics is not merely an incidental, parallel development alongside recognition theory's ascendancy. Rather, the two work seamlessly together to reorient the project from its original Marxist-Weberian paradigm (Thompson, 2016). The recognition approach decentres anti-capitalist class politics as it serves to obscure market logics and downplays their primacy in social reproduction (Fraser and Honneth, 2001; Thompson, 2016). Resultantly, there is less of a Critical Theoretical investment in engaging with the market as a primary sight of analysis for social pathologies.

Monistic recognition accounts recenter the focus of the Critical Theoretical endeavour to the cognitive capacities essential for, and the moment of, intersubjective praxis. This represents an unabashed retreat from a focus on structural-systemic logics. For McNay, this is indicative of the 'new constellation of political culture… (in which) … the centre of gravity has shifted from redistribution' (McNay, 2008: 89). Recall that for Honnethian recognition theorists 'even distributional injustices must be understood as the institutional expression of social disrespect – or, better said, of unjustified relations of recognition' (Fraser and Honneth, 2001: 114). From such an optic the dynamics of market forces must be construed as epiphenomenal to an antecedent recognition order. Political-economy is consumed by the primal dyadic relationship (McNay, 2008). When the recognition lens is presented as capable of scoping the entirety of social reality, the utility of placing political-economy at the centre of one's analysis is obviously limited.

The propensity to view 'society as a network of recognition relations' (Fraser and Honneth, 2001: 212) has led to the 'displacement' of political economic concerns at 'precisely the moment when an aggressively expanding neoliberal capitalism is radically exacerbating economic inequality' (McNay, 2008: 92). To the extent that recognition theoretical approaches serve to displace and decenter political economy, one must view Honnethian approaches as complicit in the prevailing 'neoliberal amnesia' (Fraser and Honneth, 2001: 198). That Honneth, current director of the Institute for Social Research, champions an approach which serves to 'represses the critique of political economy' is remarkable (Fraser and Honneth, 2001: 198). With Honneth submitting that the very institutions of the market 'can be understood as ... [furthering] institutionalized relation(s) of mutual recognition' (Honneth, 2014b: 208), Thompson may legitimately question whether today's Critical Theory does more to 'inculcate conformity to the prevailing reality' (Thompson, 2016: 1), rather than to advance radical political praxis.

A Collision Course for Progressive Politics

In an extensive, and sometimes heated exchange with Iris Marion Young, Fraser articulated a second, equally potent, political critique of the socio-political formations precipitated by theories of recognition. Critical of Young's (1990) *Justice and the Politics of Difference*, Fraser constructed a four-fold typology of political action (Fraser, 1995a). Socio-political movements sit on two axes; of recognition or redistribution, and of affirmation or transformative intent to social structures. Movements may seek social-structural transformation to remedy distributive injustice, or may, in their mode of engagement, inadvertently, or deliberately, affirm the social-structure in their campaigns (Fraser, 1995a. 1995b). The very same applies equally to recognitive concerns. Fraser is critical of Young's work for presenting 'a brief for affirmative recognition', without ever submitting how her theory can lead to 'transformative redistribution' (Fraser, 1995b). Fraser contends that the optimum configuration would be a transformative agenda which incorporates both redistributive and recognitive concerns. In contrast to this ideal, Fraser submits that recognition politics has an in-built tendency to further restrictive affirmative politics which can be counterproductive to the transformative goals of more radical progressive movements.

What is essential here is that Fraser (1995a, 1995b) submits that recognition based political movements have an inbuilt affinity to develop in a manner which is affirmative of broader social structures. This is not to state that all recognition-based political movements will become reactionary, nor that they will all stifle more radical progressive causes. Fraser's position is more measured, simply arguing there is a proclivity in recognition-centred campaigns to such a development. As Fraser has advanced elsewhere (Fraser and Honneth, 2001), recognition-based theorisations serve to occlude the significance of market logics. As a result, the politics of recognition has inevitably become more about status and identity, as Young (1990) admits to. Obvious examples of such 'affirmative' recognition campaigns could be reservation, affirmative action, or marriage equality. Such campaigns, in their desire to end a form of discrimination within a particular social order, seek not the abolition of the social order itself, but rather a better accommodation for a class of people within it. They are thus easily co-opted by neoliberal interests, draining them of any transformative intent. Drucker (2011) paints exactly such a development with the gay-rights movement, which he claims has 'fractured' under neoliberal capitalism. Brighton Pride, for instance, perhaps the epitome of a contemporary recognition-political moment, used to be a radical, transformative project, concerned with welfare provision and socialist transition. Today, Pride marchers follow under the banner of the event's lead patron: American Express (Wilson, 2018).

Once such events have developed a clear 'affirmative' politics, Fraser (1995a, 1995b) argues that they may inadvertently directly impede other progressive movements which seek more radical social-structural transformation. This is not merely a problem of displacement: of transformative ideals being left behind by a move to recognition politics. Rather, while different progressive groups seek both 'affirmative recognition' and 'transformative distribution' at the same moment, we witness the real occurrence of progressive causes unnecessarily impeding each other. It is of course possible for the same political actor to believe in two, or more, entirely non-mutually excluding, political causes: racial equality and social democracy, for instance. What is highly problematic, with the ascent of affirmative recognition politics, is that the same political actor may, through supporting a recognition affirmative movement on one day, and a transformative socialist movement on the other, be impeding their own political objectives.[33]

---

[33] Fraser (1995a) discusses a case of a black rights march in New York City, where, to her incredulity, nearly a million people marched through Wall Street without a single anti-capitalist banner. The demand for better inclusion within the capitalist system was, for her, clearly affirming the political-economic structure: the demand is merely for better inclusion within it. For Fraser, a marcher X, who, the very next day, marched in protest against the neoliberal order, would have been affirming the structure one day, attempting to transform it the next. While Fraser's characterisation of race based movements as affirmative is debatable, the problematic she poses is convincing. To this extent *Black Lives Matter* seeks an explicitly transformative, rather than an affirmative politics (Ransby, 2015).

Conclusion

This chapter has argued that Honneth's recognition-theoretical approach is problematic social-theoretically, philosophically and politically. As the dominant approach to engaging with social pathologies draws heavily from Honneth's Critical Theory of Recognition this is a serious impediment to radical pathology diagnosing social critique.

The first section of the chapter offered a social-theoretical argument. Here I argued that an exclusively recognition derived account of the social serves to exclude numerous species of social pathologies from view as the social world cannot be engaged with solely as a recognition order: it is much more complex than that. Drawing on Fraser, I demonstrated how numerous social logics (for example, those of capital) must be theorised as more than mere extrapolations of recognition dynamics. Next, I argued that the very desire to frame the entirety of the social through a singular optic was problematic and unnecessary. In contrast, I reiterated how this thesis champions a 'polycentric' and 'multilateral' approach to Critical Theory (Fraser and Honneth, 2001).

The second section focused on the philosophical weaknesses of Honneth's approach. This discussion served to introduce Thompson's *Domestication of Critical Theory*, an important intervention, and a text which be returned to repeatedly in this thesis. Here, I drew out how the dominant recognition approach falls victim to what Thompson (2016) presents as the neo-Idealist fallacy. I argued that Honneth's recognition-theoretical approach can thus be considered to be based on an unjustifiably idealist social ontology, and echoed Bollenbeck's (2019) stinging indictment: that Honneth succeeded in turning Hegel on his head … and back again. This section further criticised the universalist pretensions of Honneth's account: drawing on McNay (2008) and Fanon I argued that the idea that there is a singular intersubjective struggle that occurs universally is doubtful considering the experiences of coloniality. Finally, in this section, through an engagement with Celikates (2018), I assessed the recognition-theoretical claim to have solved the 'theory-immanent' problem.

The last section of this chapter engaged with the political arguments against Honneth's recognition-theoretical approach. Drawing on Thompson, I argue how a recognition theoretical approach, non-incidentally, furthers an erasure of capital critique. Finally, through an engagement with the Fraser-Young debate I echoed Fraser's concerns with the ascent of recognition affirmative political movements which could bring progressive activists into direct conflict, potentially with themselves: standing upon the American Express banner at the front of Brighton Pride one afternoon, then picketing against big-capital the next.

The arguments in this chapter are submitted to support my primary social-theoretical intervention: destabilising the ascendant, recognition-derived approach to social pathology diagnosing critique. My thesis proper argues for the need for Critical Theory urgently to return to a differentiated, not solely recognition based, understanding of 'social pathology'. To reiterate, the central submission of my thesis is that a crucial resource of Critical Theory, the diagnosis of social pathologies, is increasingly being rendered impotent through its troubling and unnecessary marriage with Honneth's restrictive recognition approach. While the diagnosis of social pathologies previously provided a potent social theoretical framework, which united the interdisciplinary Critical Theoretical project (Chapter One), today 'pathology diagnosis' is increasingly viewed through an exclusively 'pathologies of recognition' or 'recognition-cognitive' lens (Chapter Three).

Chapter Three

Recognition Theory and Social Pathology: A Troubling Marriage[34]

Having outlined the limitations of the dominant recognition-derived approach to conducting social theory (Chapter Two), I now address how such a framing impacts social pathology scholarship. In contrast to the plurality of traditions which undergird pathology diagnosing critique (Chapter One, Chapters Four-Six), this thesis argues that a limited, recognition-derived understanding of social pathology, is increasingly dominant. This transition has impeded the potency of the pathology diagnosing approach and should be understood as contributing to the 'domestication' of Critical Theory more broadly (Thompson, 2016). Chapter Three thus makes an important contribution to my broader argument by charting the ascendancy of recognition-derived framings of social pathology across the Critical Theoretical literature.

This chapter is comprised of four sections. First, I examine the rise of the 'pathologies of recognition' approach to Critical Theory, which is closely tied to Honneth's Critical Theory of Recognition (as critiqued in Chapter Two). This discussion engages with the 'Jyväskylä School' and touches on what might be deemed a protean 'Essex School' of social pathology. The second section engages with Honneth's (2014) problematic framing of 'misdevelopments' [*Fehlentwicklungen*] within *Freedom's Right*. While Honneth appears to have discarded this framing in his more recent work, it is worth engaging with as it serves to complicate the discussion on social pathology (Freyenhagen, 2015) and furthers the ascent of recognition-derived social criticism (Schaub, 2015). The third section outlines the ascent of a particularly restrictive, 'recognition-cognitive' approach to engaging with social pathologies. This framing was precipitated by a reading of Honneth's approach to social pathology offered by Zurn (2011). While all three of these developments have served to 'domesticate' the diagnosis of social pathologies, I argue that the 'recognition-cognitive' framework has had the greatest impact in the contemporary literature and should be viewed as the most restrictive and most 'domesticating'. Having outlined my criticisms of the dominant recognition-derived approaches to social pathology scholarship, section four predicts, and responds to possible rejoinders that might be offered from supporters of the dominant approaches to social pathology diagnosing critique.

While this chapter underscores the excessively cognitive nature of Zurn's framing, an important distinction needs to be drawn between Zurn's approach and antecedent

---

[34] Approximately 1200 words of this chapter, specifically my critique of Zurn's framing of social pathology, has been published as part of my article in the *European Journal of Social Theory* 22(1): 45-62, Harris N (2019) Recovering the Critical Potential of Social Pathology Diagnosis.

understandings of social pathology. While many of the conceptions of social pathology championed in later sections of this thesis have a cognitive dimension, none are *exclusively* cognitive. The cognitive impediment described by Rousseau (Chapter Four), Hegel (Chapter Five) or Fromm (Chapter Six) is but one part of the pathology; *a companion to, or manifestation of, pathologies in the manifest social world* (Strydom, 2011). The ascendant recognition-cognitive framing focuses solely on pathologies located 'in the head' of the social subject, negating the social dynamics existing in the material world (Freyenhagen, 2015: 136). My thesis contends this has undeniably 'domesticating' consequences for pathology diagnosing critique.

The Ascent of the Pathologies of Recognition Framework

With research programmes[35] and special issues[36] increasingly marching under the 'Pathologies of Recognition' banner, it is evident that the contemporary study of social pathology has developed a distinctly recognitive inflection (Hirvonen and Pennane, 2019; Schaub and Odigbo, 2019, *inter alia*). Honneth's scholarship, particularly his Critical Theory of Recognition, is of unparalleled importance in shaping contemporary discussions on social pathology (and Critical Theory more broadly) (Laitinen, Särkelä and Ikäheimo, 2015; Thompson, 2016, 2017, 2019). Perhaps the most provocative intervention provided by Honneth's Critical Theory of Recognition is his submission that a sufficiently well-ground recognition lens can provide a singular optic through which to examine and critique the social totality (Honneth, 1995; Fraser and Honneth, 2003, *inter alia*; as critiqued in Chapter Two). Honneth's Critical Theory is further distinct in that it holds recognition as the 'fundamental overarching' social category and views all other logics and modalities as 'derivative' (Fraser and Honneth, 2001: 3). While the ascendance of such critical theories of recognition has led to an increasingly divided academy (Fraser, 1995; McNay, 2008; Thompson, 2016), the dominant literature on social pathology remains overwhelmingly recognition-centric (Canivez, 2011; Hirvonen, 2015; Laitinen, Särkelä and Ikäheimo, 2015). While Honneth has an impressive theoretical output on both social pathology (2000, 2004, 2007a, 2007b, 2014, *inter alia*) and on recognition (1995, 2008, 2014 *inter alia*; Fraser and Honneth, 2001) it is the 'Jyväskylä School' that truly united these theoretical concerns (Laitinen, 2015).[37]

---

[35] See, for example, Arto Laitinen's work as part of the Academy of Finland's project entitled 'Pathologies of Recognition'.
[36] See, for example, *Studies in Social and Political Thought*. 2015 Vol. 25(1).
[37] It is curious to note that Honneth himself does not utilise the language of 'pathologies of recognition' despite providing the central theoretical 'ingredients' across his research interests.

The Importance of the Jyväskylä School for furthering a pathologies of recognition approach

It was within the Finnish academy that the fusion of Honneth's otherwise siloed concerns of 'pathology' and 'recognition' were united, both in social theory and social research. Indeed, if one makes any engagement with the literature on 'pathology' or 'recognition' it is hard to escape the 'Jyväskylä school' (Laitinen, Särkelä and Ikäheimo, 2015: 24). This group has published extensively as individuals and as a collective, with key figures including Arto Laitinen, Heikki Ikäheimo and Arvi Särkelä. Despite their moniker the academics who comprise this 'school' are spread beyond Jyväskylä, hence the increasing impact of their paradigm across international scholarship.[38] Through various research projects, conferences, and with a focused doctoral and postdoctoral community, academics across *The University of Tampere* and *The University of Jyväskylä* have published an extensive array of books, paper and book-chapters, furthering recognition scholarship and its intertwinement with social pathology.[39]

There are three features typical of the Jyväskylä School's approach to diagnosing social pathologies, all of which can be traced to Honneth's Critical Theory of Recognition: a) a restrictively recognition-derived approach to social pathologies, b) an attempt to theorise social pathologies that effect both isolated individuals and broader groups through the recognition lens, and c) a commitment to both social theory and social research utilising the 'pathologies of recognition' framework.

Hirvonen's (2015, 2019) research is indicative of the Jyväskylä's School's 'pathologies of recognition' approach. Hirvonen views social pathologies as being, definitionally, 'failures of realizing recognition relationships successfully' (Hirvonen, 2015: 209). From such a position, the role of the critical social theorist becomes simply analysing pathologies of recognition, the intersubjective disconnects responsible for failed recognition relationships (Hirvonen, 2015: 209). True to Honneth's Critical Theory of Recognition, if the entirety of the social world can be understood through a recognition approach, why would critical social theorists desire to look for pathologies elsewhere? In this regard, the Jyväskylä school shows a remarkable fidelity to Honneth's unifocal Critical Theory. The problem, as established in Chapter Two, is that Honneth's approach is fatally flawed and 'domesticating' (Fraser and Honneth, 2001; McNay, 2008; Thompson, 2016). As Hirvonen's definition of social pathology (above) indicates, for Jyväskylä school theorists, social pathologies are solely to be understood as 'pathologies of recognition'. For Laitinen and Ikäheimo (2011), this reflects both the foundational nature of

---

[38] Laitinen, Särkelä and Ikäheimo claim that there are academics operating as part of the 'Jyväskylä School' in locations as diverse as Tampere, Sydney, Frankfurt, Lucerne, St. Gallen and Helsinki (2015: 24). In the four years since they submitted this the impact of their approach and its critical research has grown further.
[39] Recognition and Social Ontology etc

recognition relationships as advanced by Honneth's *Critical Theory of Recognition*, but also a distinct commitment to a social ontology which places supreme importance on the recognition moment. For Laitinen and Ikäheimo, both the socially produced nature of our understanding of 'being', and the 'being that is the social', can be best understood through a recognition perspective. One could state that the Jyväskylä school, like Honneth, is 'recognition down to the core': for such theorists no other perspective is necessary.

For the Jyväskylä school, recognition is not merely of utility to explain the pathologies of the ideal-typical subject-meets-subject recognition moment; the so-called 'intersubjective dyad'. Rather, in keeping with Honneth (1995) and Martineau, Meer and Thompson (2012), the recognition approach can be adapted to productively explain broader group dynamics (Hirvonen, 2015). For Hirvonen, it is entirely possible to 'map out and analyze pathologies of collective recognition' (Hirvonen, 2015: 210), and, through doing so, to outline the 'systemic and institutional problems in providing opportunities for flourishing lives' (Hirvonen, 2015: 209). In his more recent scholarship, Hirvonen (2019) has focused on the ascent of populist discourses and political campaigns, analysed through the pathologies of recognition approach. Such an understanding explicitly contends that the recognition paradigm is well placed to outline the pathologies intrinsic to social structural logics which impact on collectives. In such an analysis one can hear the resounding echo of Honneth's exclusively recognition approach to the social, as outlined in his debate with Fraser (Fraser and Honneth, 2001). As stated in the previous chapter, such an approach is untenable.

Finally, it is worth stressing how the Jyväskylä school has further entrenched the pathologies of recognition approach by utilising the perspective to conduct social research. While O'Neill and Smith's edited collection *Recognition Theory as Social Research* (2012) laid the foundations for social research conducted through a 'pathologies of recognition' approach, there was no explicit engagement with the framing of 'pathology' in their collection. Yet again, it is the Jyväskylä school who unite 'pathologies' and 'recognition'. For example, Niemi (2015) uses an explicitly 'pathologies of recognition' framing for his research into social work. As with the Jyväskylä school's social theory, such an approach has proved popular and impacted other research collectives. For instance, Houston and Montgomery (2017) utilise an explicitly 'pathologies of recognition' approach to 'reflect critically on contemporary social pathologies' that pose challenges to 'critical and radical social work'. For the social researchers and social theorists of the Jyväskylä school, and those who draw upon their approach, recognition is of supreme, overarching importance to understanding social pathologies. To summarise in their own words, they view their research as seeking to

... critically compliment the Hegel-inspired picture outlined by Honneth and others following him of successful relationships of recognition and their generally optimistic conception of the content, dynamics and results of needs, demands and struggles for recognition with an account of denied, lacking or rejected recognition (Laitinen, Särkelä, Ikäheimo, 2015: 5).

Beyond the Jyväskylä School

Drawing upon Honneth, and the foundations laid by the Jyväskylä school, a plurality of theorists extend the Honnethian approach to its logical conclusions: arguing that the recognition paradigm can be drawn upon to identify *all* social pathologies (Zurn, 2011; Canivez, 2011; Fraser and Honneth, 2011; see Freyenhagen 2015; Thompson 2016, 2019; Canivez, 2019). Schaub and Odigbo's (2019) paper 'Expanding the Taxonomy of (Mis-)Recognition in the Economic Sphere' epitomises this approach. One could perhaps go as far to tentatively state Schaub is part of a protean 'Essex School' of social pathology scholarship.[40]

The distinguishing feature of such an approach is the counter-intuitive attempt to utilise the 'pathologies of recognition' framing to engage with explicitly market logics.[41] Schaub and Odigbo (2019) argue that by locating 'need' within the framing of 'recognition', the pathologies of the market can be comprehended in an 'expanded taxonomy' through the recognition paradigm. Through outlining the 'consumptive' and 'productive' facets in recognition of need, esteem and respect, the co-authors urge social pathology theorists to engage with the 'variants of misrecognition that ... [form] part of the economic sphere' (Schaub and Odigbo, 2019: 117). From such a perspective, those who 'have to rely on food and clothes banks' are victim of 'consumptive need misrecognition' (Schaub and Odigbo, 2019: 112). To those outside the recognition-paradigm, such an approach will surely raise an eyebrow at the very least because it seems such an unnatural framing.[42] Scepticism as to the utility of such an approach may be further aroused due to two facets of the co-author's framework.

First, as the co-authors stress, their intervention is solely designed to enhance and polish the recognition approach. There is no attempt to see how recognition could be connected to, or utilised alongside, other framings of social pathology. Their key argument is that an

... expanded taxonomy is a useful tool for social pathology theorists, who should appreciate the full range of variants of misrecognition when diagnosing pathologies of misrecognition in the economic sphere (Schaub and Odigbo, 2019: 103).

---

[40] Fabian Freyenhagen, Jörg Schaub and Timo Juetten, all based at the University of Essex, have published extensively on recognition, and have connected it to social pathology in varying ways throughout their research. The claim they represent a 'school' is perhaps more contentious as Freyenhagen appears at best ambivalent towards the 'pathologies of recognition' paradigm, while Schaub (2019 *inter alia*) and Juetten (2017 *inter alia*) are clear proponents of the recognition-derived approach.

[41] Perhaps the most obvious reason this is counter-intuitive is because the market, not being a conscious subject, is incapable of granting recognition in any ways similar to the intersubjective praxis of the Hegelian dyad.

[42] See footnote 7.

Note that the co-authors talk of 'social pathology theorists', which would obviously include those interested in the full breadth of the pathology framework, yet immediately juxtapose this with 'diagnosing variants of misrecognition'. The sentence does not allow that social pathology theorists might invested in looking at a plurality of alternate framings of social pathology. Schaub and Odigbo represent an approach to social pathology scholarship which appears solely invested in recognition.

Second, the co-authors do not engage with the plurality of arguments against the recognition-derived approach to social pathology. There is one solitary sentence in a footnote which states that 'many argue that other systemic factors not reducible to issues related to recognition also shape outcomes in the economic sphere' (Schaub and Odigbo, 2019: 118). It is interesting that the co-authors consider there to be 'many' academics opposed to a restrictive recognition account, however they make no engagement with their arguments in the body of their text. More interestingly still, the co-authors do not even offer a single sentence stating that there are many academics who philosophically oppose the recognition derived approach (recall Chapter Two).[43] Thompson (2016), Fraser (Fraser and Honneth, 2001) and McNay (2008) all present widely read critiques of the Honnethian recognition approach which provide a critique of the ontological assumptions central to the recognition account. The co-authors' do not even offer a sentence stating this fact, let alone engaging with such arguments. This is highly indicative of the fractured nature of the academy when it comes to conversations surrounding social pathology.

To stress, this analysis has not been offered to single out Schaub and Odigbo for special treatment: on the contrary, I turn to their paper as it is indicative of the siloed and contested nature of recognition theoretical engagements with social pathology more broadly (Freyenhagen, 2015; Thompson, 2016, 2019; Canivez, 2011, 2019). What the discussion here has begun to draw out is that both within and beyond the Jyväskylä School there is a literature which marries recognition and social pathology. Crucially, this fusion occurs in such as a way as to obscure alternate framings of social pathology.

On Misdevelopments

It is worth engaging with the framing of social 'misdevelopments' which Honneth (2014) presents in *Freedom's Right*. This can be read as a further factor fusing recognition and social

---

[43] I read this brief footnote as admitting to a knowledge of the social-theoretical critiques of recognition theory, which are largely centred around the criticism that the recognition approach fails to capture the full range of social pathologies (see Chapter Two).

pathology (Schaub, 2015: 113).[44] Following Freyenhagen (2015), I argue Honneth's addition needlessly complicates the discussion on social pathology and is unworkable. Yet, more importantly than the failure of the intervention, I argue Honneth's turn to 'misdevelopments' is indicative of the trend to 'domesticate' the diagnosis of social pathologies. Honneth is clear that he considers obstacles to social freedom not to be 'social pathologies' but 'misdevelopments'. Honneth's intervention here attempts to arbitrarily restrict the purview of social pathology.

Honneth's framing of misdevelopments in Freedom's Right

Honneth's *Freedom's Right* marks his greatest investment in 'misdevelopments' as pertaining to a social malady distinct from 'social pathologies' (Freyenhagen, 2015: 143). It is essential to acknowledge the idiosyncratic nature of *Freedom's Right*. The text unites a methodological commitment to normative reconstructionism with investments in recognition theory, and a reconceptualised (metaphysically absent) Hegelianism. In lieu of Hegel's metaphysics, Honneth sporadically champions an Apel inspired hermeneutic-discursive hybridity.[45] It is within the horizon of such a rich and multifaceted project that Honneth distinguishes between 'social pathologies' and 'misdevelopments', which perhaps might help explain the lack of clarity on this particular thematic. To be charitable to Honneth, *Freedom's Right* has lots of things 'going on', and this certainly isn't his main theoretical investment. That said, Honneth attempts to provide clarity to the distinction. 'Social pathologies' are held to be the obstacles preventing legal and moral freedom;

> Social embodiments of misinterpretations for which the rules of action themselves are at least partially responsible (Honneth, 2014b: 128).

In contrast, misdevelopments are the obstacles held to be preventing 'social freedom', and thus,

> must be sought elsewhere, not in the constitutive rules of the respective system of action (Honneth, 2004: 129).

Schaub helps differentiate between the two:

> Let me give you an example for each [misdevelopments and social pathologies]: the socially triggered tendency to withdraw from communicative relationships and to view one's involvements with others almost exclusively from the impersonal standpoint of law is one of Honneth's examples of a legal pathology. Think, for instance, of a husband who, anticipating his divorce, starts to evaluate each and every move he makes strategically according to how it will be evaluated by a judge who has to decide on the custody of the couple's children. The deregulation of the market sphere can serve as an

---

[44] Schaub (2015: 113) writes that 'Honneth associates different types of social aberrations [pathologies and misdevelopments] with the two types of relationships of recognition.' One must note that for Schaub, who is entirely recognition-centric in his scholarship, this analysis may not be seen as intentionally furthering a recognition-theoretical approach.

[45] For a full discussion on the methodological strengths and limitations of *Freedom's Right* see the special issue of *Critical Horizons* 16(2).

example of a social misdevelopment. For it leads to a situation in which interactions between individuals are less and less about general and reciprocal interest satisfaction (Schaub, 2015: 113).

Despite a lack of clarity in the broader literature, two comments can be made with some certainty: (a) central to Honneth's distinction between 'social pathologies' and 'misdevelopments' is whether the identified social malady serves as an obstacle to the development of 'legal' or 'moral' freedom (pathologies) or to 'social' freedom (misdevelopments), and (b) the obstacles to the attainment of social freedom are, for Honneth, not due to problems intrinsic to the social logics itself, but to a deviation from their harmonious, emancipatory potential.

The troubling development of 'misdevelopments'

Freyenhagen's (2015) paper 'Honneth on Social Pathologies: A Critique' is rightly scathing about Honneth's framing of 'misdevelopments', which is deemed fundamentally 'unworkable' (Freyenhagen, 2015: 131). Similar to Schaub (2015), but with a subtly distinct emphasis, Freyenhagen understands the distinction Honneth attempts to make between 'pathologies' and 'misdevelopments' as based on whether the social malady is due to 'internal' factors with the sphere of freedom (pathologies) or 'external' factors, which serve to retard the inherent emancipatory potential of a social sphere (misdevelopments) (Freyenhagen, 2015: 146-147).

Freyenhagen rightly critiques the distinction on two grounds. Firstly, it is unclear why certain social maladies might not be both 'misdevelopments' and 'pathologies' simultaneously, a consideration Honneth's theoretical infrastructure in *Freedom's Right* seems unable to accommodate (2015: 147). Second, the idea that social freedom does not have any pathologies seems arbitrary and unjustifiable:

> social freedom – roughly modelled on the idea of love, such that the pursuit and realization of your ends is reciprocally implied in the pursuit and realization of my own ends, and vice versa is not just a superior freedom which provides the proper framework and the preconditions for the other two, but is so innocent and pure just like love is often thought to be that it can never be at fault when things go wrong within its practices and institutions. In this way, misdevelopments are reserved for the practices of social freedom, and only legal and moral freedom's deviations are due to their internal structure (Freyenhagen, 2015: 147).

As Freyenhagen argues, this distinction is never fully justified by Honneth, and is ultimately arbitrary and unhelpful. Freyenhagen goes so far as to identify thirteen 'misdevelopments' within *Freedom's Right* which fail to neatly fit into Honneth's parameters: some overlap between being obstacles to legal, moral and social freedom, others are simply underdeveloped or contradictory. Some are perhaps better considered as 'injustices' or 'illegitimacies'

(Freyenhagen, 2015: 148). This serves to transition Critical Theoretical critique away from its more foundational, deeper questions.

Yet the clear theoretical limitations of Honneth's framework are not the main concern of this chapter. What is of more interest to me is how recent developments in social pathology scholarship have served to restrict the potency of the framing and have fused social pathology with recognition. In this regard, Honneth's framing of misdevelopments is crucially domesticating as it serves to restrict the framing of social pathologies, and to remove central social-structural logics from its purview. As Freyenhagen states,

> ... A number of social problems that prior to Freedom's Right were counted by Honneth as social pathologies ... have now become misdevelopments. This might seem to be merely a rebranding of them. However ... reframing these problems as misdevelopments suggests that the sphere in which they occur – the market – and its associated norms are itself unproblematic and should merely be protected from external influences (rather than overcome or at least contained in virtue of an in-built tendency to generate social pathologies). The sphere and its norms are removed from critical view, with a sole emphasis of critique on external influences (Freyenhagen, 2015: 148).

Returning to Thompson's (2016) critique of 'domesticated' Critical Theory, such a move away from the focus on central social logics, such as the market, previously of fundamental concern to Critical Theory, is a clear 'domestication'. For Thompson, an analysis of the logics which 'pulse beneath the surface' (Thompson, 2016: 7) of capitalist society needs to be at the core of Critical Theory. In *Freedom's Right,* Honneth's turn to the language of 'misdevelopments' serves to make this concern inaccessible to social pathology diagnosing critique. Honneth's desire is clear, to restrict the purview of 'social pathology' to instances where the individual fails to realise the emancipatory potentials for recognition within the legal and moral spheres of freedom (Schaub, 2015). That the director of the Institute of Social Research would advocate a framing of social theory which excludes the central logics of social reproduction (capitalist logics) from critique would be unthinkable to first- and second-generation Critical Theorists. Honneth's framing of misdevelopments, and his desire to move market logics into a terrain which can never evince social pathologies, evinces the truly 'domesticated' nature of contemporary Critical Theory (Thompson, 2016).

The ascendancy of the recognition-cognitive conception of social pathology

Zurn's second-order disconnect framework

The contemporary discussion on social pathology was significantly influenced by Christopher Zurn's intervention which served to: (a) both (further) fuse pathology diagnosis with recognition, and (b) restrict the framing to a recognition-cognitive model (Freyenhagen, 2015). Zurn argued that social pathologies 'exhibit a similar underlying conceptual structure, that of second-order disorders' (Zurn, 2011: 345). Such disorders operate through a

> ... fundamental disconnect between first-order contents and the subjects' reflexive grasp of the origins and character of those contents, where that gap systematically serves to preserve otherwise dubious social structures and practices (Zurn, 2011: 348).

Zurn's framing of social pathology is considerably closer to a structure that one would traditionally associate with ideology, and he indeed argues that,

> Marx's articulation of a theory of ideology .... is a good example of the conceptual structure ... central to Honneth's attempts to reinvigorate the practice of social critique through the diagnosis of social pathologies: namely, the grasp of social pathologies as second-order disorders (Zurn, 2011: 346).

For Zurn, ideology represents an archetypal social pathology insofar as

> it contributes to deleterious social outcomes through a kind of second-order disorder, a disorder socially patterned and thereby contributes to unwanted social outcomes (Zurn, 2011: 348).

While straightforward factual inaccuracies which can inhibit self-realisation (for instance, believing that Cambridge is the capital of England) can arise from plain mistakes, or miscommunication, ideological beliefs can only be 'explained by second-order distortions in the process of belief-formation and stabilisation' (Zurn, 2011: 347-8). It is only maladies of this second species that Zurn holds as social pathologies. For Zurn, all social pathologies are thus cognitive impairments where second-order operations are impeded, precipitating undesired social outcomes. It is immediately apparent that Zurn's conception of social pathology is radically cognitivist.

Zurn must also be credited with explicitly marrying this cognitivist framing with Honneth's critical theory of recognition. It is Zurn's intervention which moved social pathology scholarship in both a cognitivist and a recognition-theoretical manner. It is this particular conception of social pathology that I term 'recognition-cognitive'. As Zurn establishes, in his framework, it is ideological acts of recognition which represent the reality of social pathologies.

> Honneth seeks a way of identifying, in the act of the recognition relationship itself, which markers we could use to say that it is an ideologically distorting, rather than a socially productive, instance of interpersonal recognition. His answer is basically that acts of recognition are ideological when there is a substantial gap between the evaluative acknowledgement or promise that the act centres upon, and the institutional and material conditions necessary for the fulfilment of that acknowledgement or promise (Zurn, 2011: 349).

From Zurn's perspective, deficient recognition relationships alone can no longer be framed as social pathologies. As Zurn argues, 'without the second-order disorder, what we might generically call 'bad' acts of recognition (misrecognition, non-recognition) are not ideological', therefore for Zurn, they 'cannot count as social pathologies' (Zurn, 2011: 349). This brings us to an understanding of social pathologies as socially induced second-order cognitive disconnects which perpetuate ideologically structured recognition relationships. The comparatively restrictive nature of this conception is immediately obvious, and has been subjected to critical analysis (Freyenhagen, 2015; Laitinen, 2015).

Freyenhagen rightly comments that Zurn's formulation serves to locate social pathologies solely 'in the head' (Freyenhagen, 2015: 136). Furthering Thompson (2016), I argue the transition to Zurn's approach marks a clear 'domestication' a such a framing fails to equip social theorists with the tools essential for identifying problems existing in the broader social world; conceptual tools previously offered by the broader conceptions of social pathology (Chapter One, Chapters Four to Six). Freyenhagen reads Zurn's conception of social pathology as stating that 'the problem is how people interpret the world, not that it needs changing at a fundamental level' (Freyenhagen, 2015: 145). What Laitinen describes as the 'institutional reality' of social freedom is untouched by Zurn's characterisation (Laitinen, 2015: 44). It should be noted that while Freyenhagen and Laitinen both critique the restrictive and cognitivist nature of Zurn's framing, the heightened limitations produced by Zurn's marriage of the cognitive with the recognitive is left unaddressed in their analysis. This is perhaps because both theorists remain within a broadly 'pathologies of recognition' paradigm. It is worth noting that even for scholars who embrace the recognition-theoretical framing of social pathology, Zurn's account is seen as too restrictive. This is not because of its recognition-centricism, but because of the tight confines of its cognitive requirement.

Zurn's influence on Honneth

Despite the restrictive nature of Zurn's framing of social pathology, his account has been highly influential (Freyenhagen, 2015: 136). While Honneth does not explicitly adopt Zurn's formulation to the letter, his framing of social pathology in the preface to *The Idea of Socialism* (for example) is clearly reflective of Zurn's analysis. This is in clear contrast to Honneth's (2000, 2007) earlier framings of social pathology: consider his discussion of Rousseau and Hegel as 'social pathologists'. This increasingly cognitive understanding is reiterated by Honneth when he introduces social pathologies as being 'found at a higher stage of social reproduction' and functioning to 'impact subjects' reflexive access to primary systems of actions and norms' (Honneth, 2014b: 86). Elsewhere, Honneth explicitly utilises Zurn's framing of second-order disorders, introducing pathologies as 'deficits of rationality in which first-order beliefs and practices can no longer be acquired and implemented at a second order' (Honneth, 2014b: 86). That said, it is worth stressing that Honneth does not simply adopt Zurn's framing verbatim. Rather, his discussion leads towards social pathologies being evinced through *Verhaltenserstarrung*; a rigidity 'in social behaviour' and self-relation (Honneth, 2014b: 87).

However, in the final analysis, this rigidity is ultimately a manifestation of the second-order cognitive disconnect articulated by Zurn.

Returning briefly to Laitinen's critique, Honneth intentionally locates social pathologies beyond the complex 'institutional reality' of 'social freedom' (Laitinen, 2015: 44). Honneth presents social pathologies as only existing in the realms of legal and moral freedom; as stated above the maladies of 'social freedom' are presented instead as 'misdevelopments'. Thus, returning to Freyenhagen's useful turn of phrase, Honneth's *Freedom's Right* follows Zurn in locating social pathologies entirely 'in the head': as cognitive disconnects restricting subjects' capacity to realise their own moral and legal freedoms (Freyenhagen, 2015).

In his most recent work, *The Idea of Socialism*, Honneth makes limited use of the notion of social pathology. He does however turn to it in one intriguing passage:

> It might help to recall that current economic and social events appear far too complex and thus opaque to public consciousness to be capable of intentional transformation. This is particularly true when it comes to processes of economic globalisation in which transactions are carried out too quickly to be understood; here a kind of second-order pathology seems to make institutional conditions appear as mere givens, as being 'reified' and thus immune to any efforts to change them (Honneth, 2016: 3-4).

By describing the pathology as 'second order', Honneth once again lends support to Zurn's cognitive framing. What is perhaps of equal interest is that in a monograph discussing the foundational arguments in favour of socialism, Honneth does not turn again to social pathology. Considering Honneth's previous investment in the heurism, the framing of social pathology becomes conspicuous through its absence. One might infer that Honneth has perhaps become less invested in social pathology scholarship; or, as I argue, that the heurism is simply of much less utility when grasped in the restrictive recognition-cognitive manner.

The restrictive nature of the recognition-cognitive conception of social pathology

As this thesis argues, the increasing turn in the literature to recognition-derived framings of social pathology precipitates a retreat from the plurality of understandings of pathology in circulation (Chapter One, Chapters Four to Six). Not only does this approach evince the deficits expressed in Chapter Two, of debated social theoretical and philosophical robustness, the framework also excludes the critical potency harboured by rival understandings. To return to the critical animus driving social theorists to utilise pathology diagnosis critique, the diagnosis of social pathologies enables social theorists to conduct 'thicker' social criticism, probing the form of life itself (Neuhouser, 2012). As already commented (Chapter One), and as this thesis builds to establish, the critical literature presents multiple conceptions of social pathology. This breadth of interpretations enables social theorists to critique social maladies across social registers. In contrast to this rich social-theoretical tradition, the recognition-cognitive is particularly restrictive: only a set group of recognition pathologies, to Zurn, can be understood *qua* social pathologies.

The comparatively restrictive nature of the recognition-cognitive model is immediately apparent. The recognition-cognitive conception of social pathology only enabling theorists to engage with a limited, specific set of socially produced obstacles to human self-realisation. Recall in the recognition-cognitive framing only second-order disorders perpetuating ideologically structured recognition relationships are social pathologies. To pick one possible example out of many, this framework entirely excludes negative self-perpetuating dynamics, a conception of social pathology discussed by Neuhouser (2012) and seen as central to Rousseau's social pathology diagnosis (Chapter Four). This is a serious restriction on the efficacy of the framing. Such dynamics are not captured by the traditional liberal categories of injustice or illegitimacy and the framework of social pathology seems entirely apposite to describe such phenomena (Chapter One). Similarly, the conception of social pathology associated with Fromm, of pathologies of normalcy, is entirely excluded from the recognition-cognitive framework (Chapter Six). Fromm's rich contribution to the pathology diagnosing tradition placed the critique of a form of life at its centre, through its analysis of the impact of mass validation on accepted social ends and goals. The recognition-cognitive framing's inability to pose such questions further represents a 'domestication' of pathology diagnosing critique's critical potency.

It should also be noted that while the recognition-cognitive model affords a primacy to the presence of cognitive disconnects, the framing is substantially at variance from the metaphysically weighty pathologies of reason conceptualisation (Chapter Five). The left-Hegelian critique of historically effective reason enables social theorists to examine, with a singular conceptual sweep, both the cognitive capacities of subjects, and the extant development of reason within social institutions. Contrastingly, the recognition-cognitive framework focuses exclusively on the subject, and particularly, on the presence of a particular cognitive impairment. Contra the left-Hegelian tradition, the subject is not held to embody the historically unfolding developments of reason across society. Comparatively, the analytical sweep of the recognition-cognitive model is much less ambitious. Once again, one witnesses the rich social pathology diagnosing tradition being displaced by an ascendant recognition derived framing.

It is thus only the pathologies of recognition conceptualisation of social pathology that is compatible with the recognition-cognitive turn, and even then, with weighty caveats. Recall that for Zurn deficient recognition relationships that do not demonstrate a second-order disorder do not represent social pathologies. Thus, the recognition-cognitive conception of social pathology is only compatible with a subset of pathologies of recognition. As subsequent chapters shall argue, exclusively recognition-derived framings of social pathology, especially the recognition-cognitive framework, are unproductively restrictive, and serves to exclude potent, radical framings of social pathology (Chapter Four – Six).

Anticipated rejoinders and possible responses thereto

I have presented the manifold weaknesses of the Honnethian recognition-theoretical approach (Chapter Two), and demonstrated how this problematic framing has come to dominate pathology diagnosing social criticism (Chapter Three). Further, the additional limitations imposed by the Zurnian account of social pathologies as 'second-order disorders', and the domesticating impact of Honneth's framing of 'misdevelopments', have been presented and criticised (above). Having submitted my arguments against these leading approaches to pathology diagnosing social critique, it is worth briefly considering how theorists invested in such recognition-derived framings might respond. Sadly, as previously indicated, there is a worrying lack of engagement from recognition theorists with arguments against their position (Introduction; Harris, 2019). The critical literature, reflective of the broader discussion, is damagingly siloed (see my Conclusion). The following section is thus my attempt to imagine rejoinders to my criticisms, extrapolating from the limited existing scholarship to predict what recognition theorists might say if they were forced to comment on my analysis thus far.

Possible rejoinders from Honneth and/or the Jyväskylä School

In response to my critique of the pathologies of recognition framing, Honnethians, or *Jyväskylä School* theorists, might respond by reasserting the comparative merits of their position relative to prior, 'canonical' Critical Theoretical scholarship. They might stress that the pathologies of recognition framing enables Critical Theorists to move beyond the productivism of first-generation theorists (Jay, 2012: 5). In this regard, they may connect their approach to Habermasian or Gorzian insights on the dangers of productivism (Wilde, 1998: 77-83). Honneth (1995) stresses that struggles for recognition occur across social domains, not solely within the market; love and respect are equally important features of healthy intersubjective relationships.

Such an analysis could be further developed to comment on how the pathologies of recognition approach is particularly popular as a tool for engaging with irrational racial and gender hierarchies (Hirvonen, 2015), both of which were problematically peripheral in earlier Critical Theoretical scholarship (Said, 1993: 278; Allen, 2016).

On the charge of the exclusionary nature of their approach, in direct opposition to Thompson (2016), McNay (2008) and Fraser (Fraser and Honneth, 2001), Honnethians might continue to advance the position stated in *Redistribution or Recognition*: that a sufficiently well-ground recognition lens *is* capable of viewing the entirety of the social world. Despite the strength of the arguments against this position, an explicit denial seems to be the stock-response from recognition theorists. Hence, one can see Schaub and Odigbo (2019) attempting to diagnose the totality of economic pathologies through a pathologies of recognition framing, despite the voluminous literature pointing to the folly of such an enterprise (Chapter Two). For Honnethians, all that is required is a sufficiently differentiated recognition approach. If more problems are presented, the solution is to add nuance to their approach, to further finesse the recognition lens. Their contention would remain that the entirety of the social world is best understood as a network of interconnected recognition relationships and that social irrationalities are thus best characterised as deriving from pathologies of recognition (Honneth, 1995; Fraser and Honneth, 2001).

In response to the former rejoinder, that the recognition-derived approach to social pathology diagnosis, whatever its limitations, serves to overcome serious limitations in antecedent Critical Theoretical scholarship, I reply that the purported gains come at the cost of social-theoretical justifiability and political potency. While it was entirely the case that first-generation Critical Theory failed to adequately interrogate concerns of race and gender (Said, 1993; Allen, 2016), the pathologies of recognition approach fails to incorporate them into a philosophically justifiable, broader Critical Theoretical infrastructure. Further, recognition-derived approaches, in addition to displacing many of pathologies intrinsic to the economic register, and through doing so impedes the political potency of Critical Theory (Thompson, 2016), it does so without capturing the totality of the social pathologies which produce race and class hierarchies (Thompson, 2019). The goal must be to produce a Critical Theory that can incorporate an analysis of class, race and gender centred social pathologies, and for this endeavour, as this thesis argues, a 'polycentric and multilateral' engagement is required (Fraser and Honneth, 2001). The pathologies of recognition approach, while more alert to concerns of gender and race than earlier Critical Theoretical approaches, fails to provide a philosophically solid foundation for social critique, and excludes manifold social pathologies from its purview.

By presenting the entirety of the social world as a recognition order, Critical Theorists escape economism only by arriving at an unjustifiable, limited culturalism (Fraser and Honneth, 2001: Chapter One). In response, in keeping with my broader thesis, I champion the merits of a multi-perspectival pathology diagnosing account. The pathologies of recognition approach falls substantially short of such an objective.

In response to the latter rejoinder, a direct rebuttal of Thompson's (2016), McNay's (2008) and Fraser's (2001) arguments that a recognition approach cannot capture the totality of social pathologies, I point to the displaced utility of the multiple, alternate framings of social pathology (Chapters Four-Six). As I shall argue in the following chapters, a considered engagement with Rousseau, Hegel and Fromm draws out potent pathology diagnosing resources which are displaced by the dominant recognition-derived approaches to pathology diagnosing social criticism. There is a desperate need for recognition theorists to engage with the arguments against their position, as the claim that the pathologies of recognition perspective can capture the totality of the pathologies of the social world is simply unsustainable (Chapters Four-Six).

Possible rejoinders from Zurn

Similarly, Zurn, and those who identity merit in his approach (see above), might also respond to my criticisms by pointing to the relative merits of their position relative to the alternative conceptions of social pathology in wider literature. They might claim that Zurn's account provides a much-needed theoretical specificity; the 'second-order' conception of social-pathologies is much tighter, more precise than the muddle of alternate accounts of pathology in circulation (Honneth, 2007a, 2007b). They might perhaps concede that while Freyenhagen (2015) and Laitinen (2015) are correct, that the Zurnian account fails to capture the totality of insistence of social pathology found within the literature, that this exclusionary trait is in fact a strength, it sharpens the analytic focus of the heurism. The claim might be that, while there is indeed a plurality of alternate species of social wrongs not captured by their account of social pathology, Zurn's framework is advantageous in that it clearly demarcates social problems which exist at a 'higher order' of social reproduction, through its focus on the reflexive capacities' of subjects (Zurn, 2011). This conception thus succeeds in distilling the idea that there is something 'deeper', something more intrinsically wrong with the form of social life that is engaged with through the framing of social pathology (Honneth, 2000).

In response to such counter-claims, I would respond that theoretical specificity does not have to come at the cost of political impotence and social-theoretical myopia. As stated above, in keeping with Laitinen (2015), there are numerous social problems which exist, which are foundational problems for social existence, which are at least once-removed from cognitive-impairments in the social subject. The framing of social pathology has previously been utilised to provide a focus for pressing social ills which require penetrating social critique. Zurn's cognitive account removes the social-structural logics integral to capitalist society from the purview of social pathology unless that incorporate a 'second-order disorder' component. By arbitrarily excluding non-cognitive concerns from the understanding of social pathology, I would counter that Zurn's approach is theoretical unsound and politically problematic. As alternate, broader pathology diagnosing approach is essential for a more potent Critical Theory.

Conclusion

This chapter has reviewed recent developments in social pathology scholarship, charting the increasing fusion of pathology diagnosing critique and recognition theory. I have drawn out how this contingent marrying of frameworks has occurred through both the ascendancy of the 'pathologies of recognition' approach, championed by the Jyväskylä School, and through Zurn's 'recognition-cognitive' understanding. Honneth's short-lived framing of 'misdevelopments' was briefly engaged with, and the limitations of this approach were presented. By engaging with Freyenhagen (2015) and Schaub (2015), I demonstrated how Honneth's framing of 'misdevelopments' furthered the ascent of recognition theoretical approaches to social critique and attempted to displace central aspects of the pathology diagnosing tradition. Indeed, bringing Freyenhagen and Thompson (2016) into dialogue, I argued that Honneth's framing of misdevelopments serves to exclude market logics from pathology diagnosing critique: a clear domestication of Critical Theory.

While the pathologies of recognition framing needlessly restricts pathology diagnosing critique to the recognition register, I have explained how Zurn's 'recognition-cognitive' understanding enforces even more crippling restrictions. With Zurn, social pathology diagnosing critique is not merely fused with recognition theory but is further curtailed to instances of an extremely specific cognitive dynamic, to occurrences of 'second order disconnects'. Such a framing serves to drastically enfeeble the pathology diagnosing tradition.

The arguments presented here presage those of Chapters Four to Six, each of which advances the merits of an alternate, non-recognition derived framing of social pathology, which has been needlessly excluded by the dominance of recognition, and recognition-cognitive framings of social pathology.

Chapter Four

Rousseau: the social pathologist *par excellence*

Introduction

An engagement with Rousseau is essential for revitalising forms of pathology diagnosing critique which transcend the dominant recognition paradigm. This chapter presents Rousseau as the progenitor of social pathology diagnosis; and thus, in Honneth's words, as the true 'founder of social philosophy' (Honneth, 2007c: 10). Rousseau's importance for Critical Theory (Thompson, 2015; Ferrara, 2017), and indeed to sociology as a discipline more broadly, cannot be understated (Darling, 1994). Durkheim (1960) notably viewed Rousseau as the first 'sociologist'. This chapter argues that Rousseau's scholarship was dominated by his diagnosis of social pathologies (Honneth, 2007c: 7). A considered engagement with Rousseau discloses multiple, distinct framings of social pathology, which transcend the dominant recognition-derived approach (as introduced in Chapter Three).

Rousseau has also been presented as the recognition theorist *par excellence* (Neuhouser, 2008). It is therefore particularly gratifying to discover such resources within Rousseau's own work. As the secondary literature stresses, Rousseau's analysis is indeed largely concerned with the foundational 'breach of the monological self-relation' (Honneth, 2007c: 8) that led to the tragic loss of man's natural, 'pure' innocence (Darling, 1994: 6). Yet, even for Rousseau, a foundational recognition-theorist (Neuhouser, 2008), a recognition perspective, unaccompanied by alternate pathology framings, is of limited utility. This is patently evident because numerous, well-developed framings of social pathology can be found across Rousseau's *oeuvre*, which are incompatible with a 'pathologies of recognition' approach. Through a presentation of these divergent framings of social pathology, this chapter seeks to further my critique of the dominant, restrictive, recognition-derived frameworks, and to stress the plurality of potent framings of social pathology which Critical Theorists should return to.

This chapter commences with a brief reconstruction of Rousseau's *oeuvre* framed through the lens of social pathology diagnosis. This is offered to establish the true extent to which Rousseau's work was dominated by pathology diagnosing social critique. This serves to justify my contention that Rousseau, the recognition theorist *par excellence* (Shaver, 1989; Neuhouser, 2008), is equally the social pathologist *par excellence*. This analysis is also presented to justify my turn to Rousseau as a legitimate point of departure for my reconstructive project: as stressed in my introduction there was no shortage of possibilities. Such an engagement additionally serves to foreground my subsequent analysis. I contend that Rousseau's life and work can be crudely framed as:

a) 'an early Rousseau': with his initial diagnosis of social pathology,

b) 'a middle period Rousseau': with his attempts at a solution, and

c) 'a late period Rousseau': with his turn to introspective reverie as a cognitive palliative.

Having presented the centrality of 'pathology diagnosis' to Rousseau's life and work, I outline five divergent framings of social pathology which can be found within, and across, Rousseau's output. In this endeavour I both utilise, and diverge from, Neuhouser's (2012) analysis of Rousseau's *Discourse on Political Economy*. My attempt here is to present an analysis indicative of the framings of social pathology which can be located across Rousseau's work, not solely focusing on the *Discourse on Political Economy*.[46] Mine is, of course, an incomplete analysis, but serves to outline in some detail the following central pathology diagnosing framings in Rousseau's work, namely:

a) Self-perpetuating negative dynamics,

b) Unstructured dependency,

c) Cultural Pathology,

d) The colonisation of one social sphere by the logic of another, and,

e) Multiple layers of recognition pathology.

Having sympathetically introduced these multiple framings of social pathology, I move to outline three points of divergence between Rousseau's analysis and today's dominant recognition-derived framings (Chapter Three). Particular emphasis is placed on the utility of Rousseau's diagnosis of 'rationality-colonising' pathologies, the chapter argues that such an approach interfaces well with *Dialectic of Enlightenment* style arguments (Honneth, 2000). Such an approach is entirely divergent from the dominant pathologies of recognition and recognition-cognitive frameworks. Next, drawing on Neuhouser (2012), I point to the import of viewing social pathologies as being built on, or in many instances necessitating, self-perpetuating negative dynamics. As presented, such dynamics can occur without any intentional 'human malevolence' (Rousseau, 1979: 45). Indeed, *pace* the dominant recognition-cognitive framing, drawing on Rousseau, I argue that such pathologies, while ultimately experienced cognitively, are located in social practices and logics which exist at a different ontological level to that of

---

[46] Which was Neuhouser's (2012) project in 'Rousseau und die Idee einer pathologischen Gesellschaft'.

human consciousness. Echoing Neuhouser,[47] *pace* today's dominant framing of social pathology, I argue that such maladies are appropriately described in the language of pathology (Neuhouser, 2012: 637-640).

Finally, by returning to my initial exposition of Rousseau as a social pathologist, I move to reinforce the central argument of my thesis: that Rousseau himself, the father of recognition theory (Shaver, 1989; Neuhouser, 2008), turns to multiple conceptions of social pathology removed from a 'pathologies of recognition', or recognition-cognitive framework. I argue that this dramatically underscores the essential limitations of the dominant, restrictive, pathologies of recognition and recognition-cognitive frameworks. Rousseau, a crucial progenitor of recognition theory, who views the entire corruption of civilisation as precipitated by changing recognition relations, still does not attempt an analysis of the social without utilising additional, alternate, non-recognition-based framings of social pathology.

Rousseau: The consummate social pathologist

The aim of this section is to articulate how Rousseau's pathology diagnosing critique inflected his entire output, and thus to underscore the merits of my engagement with his complete corpus. This is presented to justify my turn to Rousseau as a starting point for my reconstructive project. I contend that Rousseau's diagnosis can be found in his operas, his *roman a clef*, his musicology, his plays, and his autobiography, in addition, of course, to his seminal social-theory. This section further serves to foreground my discussion of Rousseau's most prominent framings of social pathology. I present this analysis to justify my initial turn to Rousseau, rather than the legion of potential alternate scholars who have been labelled as social pathologists (Introduction; Honneth, 2007 *inter alia*). As established in my earlier chapters, I do not argue that an engagement with Rousseau alone will be sufficient to revitalise pathology diagnosing critique. Rather, as I hope to establish here, analysing his work marks an entirely appropriate place to commence such a project.

Rousseau's *oeuvre* can be crudely divided into three periods relative to his changing diagnoses of social pathology: 'an early Rousseau' (1743-1761), 'a mid-period Rousseau' (1762-1771) and 'a late Rousseau' (1772-1778). Early Rousseau is the radical pathology diagnostician, mid-period Rousseau forwarding iconoclastic palliatives, late-Rousseau, withdrawn, finding introspective means of coping with the pathologies of the social.

---

[47] While this chapter draws on Neuhouser, and approves of his analysis in 'Rousseau und die Idee einer pathologischen Gesellschaft', his broader philosophical work, such as *Rousseau's Theodicy of Self-Love* (2008) sits problematically close to the dominant recognition perspective.

The Early Rousseau: *1743-1761*

In 1750 the Academy of Dijon hosted an essay competition, inviting responses to the following stimulus: 'Has the restoration of the sciences and arts contributed to the purification of morals?' (Wokler, 2001: 23). Rousseau's submission, the famous *Discourse on the Arts and Sciences,* collected first prize, his response a resounding negative.[48] For Noone, this work marked the beginning of Rousseau's 'war with society' (Noone, 1980: 6). The *First Discourse* can be read as commencing Rousseau's lifelong investment in articulating, and, in his later work ameliorating, social pathologies.

Commencing with Horace's epigram, '*Decipimur specie recti*' (Rousseau, 1993: 3),[49] Rousseau argued that civilization is 'the bane of humanity' (Wokler, 2001: 34). Drawing on both contemporary sources and texts from antiquity, Rousseau passionately argued that society, 'maintained the appearance of all the virtues, without being in possession of one of them' (Rousseau, 1993: 5). Rousseau's indictment is that humanity has been denatured through the civilising process, leading to the erasure of mankind's 'natural', child-like innocence (Douglass, 2015). From this early stage in Rousseau's work it is the 'natural', and the 'natural world' which is triumphed, and the city which is remorselessly castigated (Lukacs, 1972: 136). Ironically, it is thus the nations which pride themselves most on their superiority in art and culture, that prove least commensurate with the conditions necessary for humankind[50] to experience their true humanity (Rousseau, 1953, 1984, 1993; Strong, 1994; Wokler, 2001). Ultimately civilisations that invest too heavily in the 'perpetual restraint' of arts driven 'society' will crumble under the weight of their supreme decadence (Rousseau, 1993: 6).

Yet despite possessing 'neither order, nor logic, nor structure' (Wokler, 2001: 23), *The First Discourse* is truly significant as a pathology diagnosing text.[51] The content of the work itself, as a social pathology, is of obvious direct relevance. *The First Discourse* offered a radical critique of the form of life, in Strong's words, it was perhaps the first essay to really show 'the homelessness'[52] of humanity (Strong: 1994: 152). Yet equally importantly for understanding Rousseau as a social pathologist is the formative influence this engagement had on his

---

[48] This text will also be referred to in this chapter as *The First Discourse.*
[49] I loosely translate this as 'we are deceived by what seems to be right'.
[50] While this project makes a concerted effort to avoid gendered pronouns and analysis more broadly, when engaging with Rousseau this is not possible. While Fromm can be translated with gender-neutral terms without impeding his analysis, Rousseau's work is explicitly gendered, to pretend to the contrary would be both obfuscating, and any such an erasure would arguably be politically problematic in itself.
[51] Rousseau himself came to dislike the *First Discourse*, regarding it 'as amongst the worst' of his writing (Rousseau, 1953: 328-9).
[52] Compare this framing with the German '*bei sich, zu Hause*' understanding of alienation [*Entfremdung*] (Hardimon, 1992: 167-8).

subsequent thinking (Damrosch, 2005). In *The Confessions*, Rousseau recalls how it was through the process of writing *The First Discourse* that he first 'saw another universe'; that he 'became a different man' (Rousseau, 1953: 327). In my analysis, it was with *The First Discourse* that Rousseau found his distinctive voice, and his identity, as a social pathologist. From this point on, all of Rousseau's published work bore (at the very least) leitmotifs of pathology diagnosis (Wokler, 2001; Damrosch, 2005): the multifarious evils of the city, the comparative majestic 'purity' of nature, the tragedies of inflamed pride, and the denaturing impact of labour in 'civilised' society.

While *The First Discourse* and *Le Devin du Village*[53] positioned Rousseau as an enigmatic contrarian, a 1753 essay, *Letter on French Music*, triggered palpable hostility from the establishment. Uniting aspects of his pathology diagnosis from *Discourse on the Arts and Sciences* with earlier fragments on musicology, Rousseau's essay earned him condemnation and infamy unprecedented in *Querelle des Bouffons*.[54] For Rousseau (1995), French music typified the pathological artificiality of the city. Northern European speech was presented as being less mellifluous, more staccato, less natural. In contrast, Southern European speech was more enchanting, more animated, more human. The inclement conditions of the 'North' precipitated a vernacular most adept for the instrumental communication of needs: 'shrill', 'unpassioned' [sic], equivalence oriented (Rousseau, 1995: 380, 407-409). The regulars of *Theatre du Palais-Royal* that Rousseau deplored were (not so) implicitly condemned for their discourse shorn of 'sweetness', suitable only for pathos-less *langue de bois* (Rousseau, 1995: 425-427). Rousseau's *Letter on French Music* is a clear continuation of the core themes of *The First Discourse*. One can image Rousseau's contempt for the forced paean to beauty cleansed for the palate of the Parisian nobility. With his contribution to the *Guerre des Bouffons* Rousseau focused his pathology diagnosing critique on the alienated, 'fraudulent', lack of humanity that the arts precipitate. Once again, it is Rousseau's voice as a social pathologist which resonates crisply throughout this essay.

While *The Discourse on the Arts and Sciences* precipitated Rousseau's rise to prominence, it was with the *Discourse on the Origins of Inequality*, four years later, that Rousseau's mature diagnosis was most memorably expressed. Retaining the pathos and interdisciplinarity of *The First Discourse*, *Discourse on the Origins of Inequality* was substantially better structured, with

---

[53] Rousseau's first successful opera, often translated as *The Village Soothsayer*. While the score is musicologically progressive, the libretto is socially conservative.
[54] *Querelle des Bouffons* (Quarrel of the Comedic Actors) is the term most often applied to the extended musicological-philosophical debate that took place in Paris between 1752-4. Sometimes known instead as *Guerre des Bouffons* (War of the Comedic Actors), the battle lines were drawn between the respective supporters of French and Italian opera.

clearer, more developed argumentation (Wokler, 2001).[55] Honneth (2007) suggests this work represents the pinnacle of Rousseau's pathology diagnosing social theory. Commencing with a fictive anthropology, Rousseau (1984) outlines how humanity has passed through three key stages: from a natural, unalienated existence, through an initial early sociality, to today's debased, pathologically alienated, social order.[56] Rousseau seeks:

> to pinpoint that moment in the progress of things when, with right succeeding violence, nature was subjected to the law; to explain by what sequence of prodigious events the strong could resolve to serve the weak, and the people to purchase imaginary happiness at the price of real happiness (Rousseau, 1984: 77-78).

In the first stage, man is initially described as a simple, self-sufficient creature:

> ... an animal less strong than some, less agile than others, but taken as a whole the most advantageously organized of all. I see him satisfying his hunger under an oak, quenching his thirst at the first stream, finding his bed under the same tree, which provided the meal; and behold, his needs are furnished (Rousseau, 1984: 81).

There existed a brief happy median, of natural but communal sociality, where humans were social but self-reliant.

> People grew used to gathering together in front of their huts or around a large tree; singing and dancing, true progeny of love and leisure (Rousseau, 1984: 114).

Yet such an idyll was not to last:

> Each began to look at others and to want to be looked at himself; he who was most handsome, the strongest, the most adroit or the most eloquent became the most highly regarded... (Rousseau, 1984: 114).

The human race began to

> ... attach importance to the gaze of the rest of the world, and ... (knew) how to be happy and satisfied with themselves (only) on the testimony of others, rather than on their own (Rousseau: 1984: 136).

Central to Rousseau's diagnosis is the rupture of man's monological self-relation. There is a foundational recognition pathology at the core of Rousseau's diagnosis (Neuhouser, 2008). With civilisation, '[n]atural pity suffered ... dilution' (Rousseau, 1984: 132) at the expense of an ascendant inflamed pride, *Amour-Propre*. The natural innocence of this hypostatised mid-period of human development was tragically displaced by the 'passions and caprices of civilized communities' (Rousseau: 1984: 83). Unalienated 'natural' man was lost with the ascendancy of the 'artificial faculties' (Rousseau, 1984: 81) prized by modernity.

The Second Discourse details how the ascent of an inflamed *Amour-Propre* precipitated relations of unstructured dependency. While 'man is weak when he is dependent' (Rousseau, 1984: 99), modernity precipitates 'universal dependence' (Rousseau, 1984: 98). Of equal import

---

[55] This text will also be referred to as *The Second Discourse*.
[56] For a more expansive, and more critical framing, see Robinson (2008).

was Rousseau's indictment of the pathological cultural apparatus which perpetuated this social conjecture. Based on falsehood, complicity and alienation,

> ... it was necessary in one's own interest to seem to be other than one was in reality. Being and appearance became two entirely different things (Rousseau, 1984: 119).

What I hope to establish here is the legitimacy of reading *The Second Discourse* as an exposition of social pathology. It was with this text that Rousseau truly became 'the first great critic of bourgeois society' (Plattner, 1979: 3), the social pathologist *par excellence*.

From 1762 Rousseau's diagnosis is gradually displaced by texts designed to explicitly facilitate political transition; to ameliorate the pathologies articulated.

The Mid-Period Rousseau: 1762-1771

Where previously the focus of Rousseau's work was on articulating a diagnosis of social pathology; from 1762 he produced explicitly political texts, which can be read as suggested 'cures' or 'palliatives' (Affeldt, 1999; Neuhouser, 2012). In 1762 Rousseau published two particularly 'incendiary' texts: *The Social Contract* and *Émile*.[57]

The Social Contract has been read as an explicit attempt to cure the ills outlined in *The Second Discourse* through a radical republicanism (Neuhouser, 2012: 628). *The Social Contract* was an attempt to structure society in such a way that:

> ... each citizen shall be at the same time perfectly independent of all his fellow citizens and excessively dependent on the republic (Rousseau, 1968a: 99).

Recall *The Second Discourse*'s critique of pathologically unstructured dependence. *The Social Contract* is an attempt to structure dependence: in Rousseau's formulation all must depend on the state. Such a polity, theoretically, would encourage a 'moral and communal existence' (Rousseau, 1968a: 85). *The Social Contract* presents the blueprint for a society capable of existing without the pathologies of dependence, and thus able to cultivate republican virtue (Rousseau, 1968a). There is a structural beauty in Rousseau's figuration in his attempt to recast *Amour-Propre* as a source of social cohesion rather than personal enmity (Neuhouser, 2008).[58] Through state-led processes of socialisation, the citizens of the hypostatized republic will come to direct their desire for recognition and pride towards their shared status as citizens of the same polity. What was once the greatest source of enmity has become the binding force for solidarity (Rousseau, 1968a; Neuhouser, 2008).

---

[57] Both were burned, despite substantial opposition from the philosophes. Voltaire famously stated that the burning of the text was one of the few things as atrocious as the writing of it (Gay, 1959).

[58] It is this structural beauty: the conversion of the fundamental 'fall' into the basis for redemption that animates Neuhouser's (2008) *Rousseau's Theodicy of Self-Love*.

Émile, in contrast, while equally political, and if anything, even more controversial, was essentially an expression of a critical pedagogy. While sections of the text advance pathology diagnosis, the core aim of the text was to present a methodology through which a child may be raised to cope with said social maladies. In keeping with *The Social Contract*, Émile's most important lessons are that man's 'weakness makes him sociable' (Rousseau, 1911: 182); that he should trust his inner sentiment, and that freedom is the ultimate end. Émile is fully aware that he 'cannot keep his wealth and his freedom' (Rousseau, 1911: 436). In keeping with Rousseau's earlier critique of the pathological nature of bourgeois culture, Emile is taught that

> ... [t]he rich think so much of ... their possessions ... not because they are useful, but because they are beyond the reach of the poor (Rousseau, 1911: 149).

'The cure' remains consistent with the lessons of *The Social Contract:* invest the general will with a true power, beyond that of any single subject.

In 1755 Paoli liberated Corsica from Genoan rule (Lear, 1870: 260). Rousseau had a pre-existing interest in Corsica, repeatedly remarking of its simplicity and freedom (Durant and Durant, 1967: 204; Damrosch, 2005: 386). On the invite of Buttafuoco, Rousseau enthusiastically set to drafting a constitution for the Mediterranean island. Rousseau's affective investment in this project cannot be underestimated. In May 1765, he declared,

> ... for the rest of my life I shall have no other interest but myself and Corsica; all other matters will be completely banished from my thoughts (Durrant, 1967: 204).

Corsica retained the simple way of life he so admired. He was truly exercised when France deposed Paoli, and destroyed the prospect of a free, rustic Corsican republic. For Damrosch, Rousseau's larger argument was 'that Corsica should resist modernization at all costs in order to preserve its primitive simplicity' (Damrosch, 2005: 387). Rousseau's *Constitutional Project for Corsica* is of real interest in that it represents a political project designed to prevent the onset of many of the social pathologies he has elsewhere diagnosed (Damrosch, 2005: 386-390).

In 1771 Rousseau wrote the last of his three main political texts, *Considerations on the Government of Poland*.[59] Confounding many readers, *The Government of Poland* is a somewhat conservative text (Durrant, 1967: 884). In Durrant's words,

> ... he advised the Poles to make no sudden changes in their constitution (Durrant, 1967: 884).

And yet traces of the early Rousseau still remain; his most strident demand is for federalisation and for opposing territorial expansion. A small republic might (with luck) defy the pathologising tendencies of modernity. This was the last of Rousseau's explicitly political works. His thought

---

[59] To today's reader, the title is slightly deceptive. Rather than 'Poland', Rousseau's proposal was for the Polish-Lithuanian Commonwealth.

had travelled many fathoms since *The First Discourse*. From the 'flights *in vacuo*' (Durrant, 1967: 884) of *The Social Contract*, *The Government of Poland* is materially anchored and short on abstraction. But what is clear throughout Rousseau's work to this point is his early development of a penetrating pathology diagnosis, to the creation of a three core political texts, seeking to vitiate such pathological conditions.

The Late Rousseau: 1772-1778

From 1772 to his death in 1778, Rousseau turned to introspection and reverie. Dissatisfied with the failure of his political works to achieve institutional traction, ostracised by high society as a whole; Rousseau's scholarship in this period marked a real change in style and intent. I frame the works of the 'late Rousseau' as typified by his efforts to come to terms with the pathological nature of society through a turn to introspection.

In addition to the hugely successful *Dialogues*, this period saw Rousseau's *Reveries of a Solitary Walker*. Rousseau's bleak frame of mind is well captured by its opening line, 'so now I am alone in the world' (Rousseau, 1979: 27). In his despair and isolation, Rousseau turned to a 'total renunciation of the [material] world' (Rousseau, 1979: 52), to psychically estrange himself from the evils of the pathological social conjecture. Seeing nothing but 'human malevolence' (Rousseau, 1979: 45) and 'universal conspiracy' (Rousseau, 1979: 44), Rousseau mourned 'the sweet liberty [he] ... had lost' (Rousseau, 1979: 50). In contrast, nature again, triumphs. It is the city which is the epitome of evil:

> I see nothing but animosity in the faces of men, and nature always smiles on me (Rousseau, 1979: 149).

In his final years Rousseau turned to nature, to his love of botany, and to quiet introspective reflection.

Throughout this brief sketch I have argued that Rousseau's scholarship was animated by his 'condemnation ... of modernity' (Plattner, 1979: 5); what I present as his diagnosis of social pathology. Rousseau was unique in consistently engaging with the 'depth of the human problem' (Cullen, 1993: 19); his political writings, operas, plays: all were inflected by his diagnosis of social pathology. It is thus unsurprising that the social-theoretical infrastructure of his legacy offers a wealth of resources which harbour the potential to revitalise contemporary social pathology diagnosis. Having justified turning to Rousseau as a legitimate point of departure for my broader project, I now turn to reconstruct the most potent and prominent framings of pathology in Rousseau's work.

Reconstructing Multiple Framings of Social Pathology in Rousseau's work

I now turn to reconstruct the most pertinent framings of social pathology in Rousseau's work. The aim of this exploration is to draw out conceptions of social pathology which transcend the artificial boundaries of the Honnethian-recognition derived approaches dominant in today's literature (Chapter Three). This section thus reconstructs no fewer than five framings of social pathology which, through their variance from the dominant recognition-derived paradigm, can provide important resources for revitalising contemporary pathology diagnosing critique. This analysis extends Neuhouser's (2012) engagement with Rousseau's *Discourse on Political Economy*, where he locates multiple framings of social pathology within that one text. While Neuhouser's analysis is of real utility, the following section has a more expansive focus, encompassing the breadth of Rousseau's corpus. I stress the engagement focuses on a range of Rousseau's publications: this section does not limit itself to Rousseau's social theory, rather, as argued above, one can read Rousseau as engaging in pathology diagnosing critique across the various genres and disciplines of his output.

Pathological Social Dynamics

A recurring framing of social pathology that can be found throughout Rousseau's work is his analysis of self-perpetuating negative dynamics. While so often writing in opposition to the spirit of his era, in this regard Rousseau's diagnosis is animated by a typical Enlightenment concern with modalities, logics and patterns (Delaney, 2009: 1). Indeed, in various texts Rousseau is perhaps best read as a theorist of 'vicious circles' (Noone, 1980: 67; Blackall, 1959: 465). I argue that a crucial aspect of Rousseau's diagnosis is his analysis of pathological logics, which, once established, can occur independent of human cognition and cyclically harm the social body (Neuhouser, 2012). I term such modalities, 'pathological social dynamics'. Once established, such logics:

> make a bad situation worse and ... once initiated, ... [are].... exceedingly difficult to break (Neuhouser, 2012: 637).

For Neuhouser (2012), such a social pathology is most clearly expressed in Rousseau's analysis of the home-land security problems of Ancient Rome in the *Discourse on Political Economy*.

> ... in order to raise . . . armies, tillers had to be taken off the land; the shortage of them lowered the quality of the produce, and the armies' upkeep introduced taxes that raised its price. This first disorder caused the people to grumble: in order to repress them, the number of troops had to be increased, and, in turn, the misery; and the more despair increased, the greater the need to increase it still more in order to avoid its consequences (c.f. Neuhouser, 2012: 637).

This is clearly a description of a social malady; such a logic is undeniably problematic for the society. Indeed, one would find it hard to imagine a life-world absent such species of social ill. As Neuhouser suggests, the classic problem of 'keeping up with the Jones'' is perhaps an equally pertinent example (Neuhouser, 2012: 640). It seems self-evident that Rousseau is not merely describing a lack of legitimacy, or merely a lack of justice with this critique. In agreement with Neuhouser, I argue that Rousseau is presenting such a dynamic as constitutive of an important form of social pathology.

While Neuhouser's (2012) article 'Rousseau *und die Idee einer „pathologischen' Gesellschaft'* focuses almost exclusively on *Discourse on Political Economy*, I argue that such pathological social dynamics are explored throughout the entirety of Rousseau's scholarship.

Indeed, perhaps Rousseau's most explicit submission of a pathological social dynamic is his analysis of the artist's relationship to society (Rousseau, 1960, 1997c; Delaney, 2009: 18). As established, this is a theme which permeates Rousseau's scholarship. For Rousseau (1960, 1997c), artists seek to shock and entice their audience with ever increasing contraventions of the social mores. The content presented thus needs to become ever more extreme, ever more debased. Today, an objectifying photograph of a female model in skimpy attire on an advertising billboard will turn few heads as commuters dash around the London Underground. Such an image would have been scandalous in the extreme just fifty years ago. To grab the citizens' attention in the twenty-first century, images must be truly explicit, truly risqué. Likewise, for Rousseau (1960, 1997c) the more the social body becomes inured to depravity in the arts, the more explicit, the more degenerate the content needs to become to hold society's interest. Hence for Rousseau, the unstructured rise of the arts represents a true problem for society. Far from suggesting an ever increasing humanity and a maturing aesthetic appreciation, the rise of the arts triggers a 'race to the bottom'. Ultimately the 'market for culture dialectically corrupts both artist and patron' (Noone, 1980: 91).

For Noone (1980), the most prominent 'vicious circle' expressed in Rousseau's *oeuvre* is that of the self-perpetuating destructive drive towards urbanisation.[60] The 'city is the symbol of just about all evils' for Rousseau; the spread of the city occurs entirely to the detriment of the countryside (Noone, 1980: 197). Again, as established above, this is a consistent theme of Rousseau's analysis: it is the beauty of Lake Leman (Rousseau, 1997b) which is lauded and the Parisian salons which are castigated. This is not merely a contingent, incidental aspect of Rousseau's critique of modernity. Rather, as with Rousseau's analysis of the dialectic between

---

[60] This may perhaps be better framed as 'rural de-population' and 'urbanisation'. In passages the two seems distinct, while in others they are broadly synonymised. This may be a translation issue, I defer to native speakers.

artist and patron, there is a particular pathological dynamic in operation, which is central to the social order. Noone draws this out well,

> The rural sector, the chief source of population, has no motive to increase itself unless it is guaranteed the fruits of its labour. Any increase in parasitic urban numbers entails a corresponding decrease of peasant surpluses through taxation. When this exploitation reaches a point where the law of diminishing returns leaves a family with no reason to enlarge itself, it merely maintains its present size. Any added increment of taxation reduces the former to subsistence level or below. When it thus becomes unprofitable to work the fields, young agriculturalists are forced off the land and into the city; further augmenting the list of parasites. A vicious circle results: the more the city grows, the less agriculture produces (Noone, 1980: 67).

Thus, Rousseau cautions his reader to remember,

> ... that the walls of towns are made only from the debris of rural houses. Every time I see a mansion being built in the capital I fancy I can see the whole countryside covered with hovels (Rousseau, 1968: 138).

The importance of nature, and the importance of the rustic simple village to Rousseau's imagination cannot be overstated (Douglass, 2015). In Lukacs' prose, it came to represent a distinct ontology, invested with the moral imperative to critique the 'growth of mechanisation, dehumanisation and reification' (Lukacs, 1972: 136).

The self-perpetuating dynamic which drives urbanisation occurs without human intention or cognition. Rousseau is not presenting a mistaken ideological belief, or a 'second-order disconnect' (Zurn, 2011: 345). Rather, pathological social dynamics occur, as Rousseau states, as seamlessly as 'between the first and last terms of a geometric progression' (Rousseau, 1968: 103). Rousseau's engagement with pathological social dynamics offers an important diagnostic tool. I shall return to discuss the true import of this framing in the final part of this chapter.

Cultural Pathology

A central component of Rousseau's diagnosis is his articulation of the pathological state of modern culture (Wokler, 2001). While this analysis is partially secondary to Rousseau's critique of unstructured dependency, it retains a central role in his theoretical infrastructure. While this aspect of Rousseau's diagnosis can be located across his work, it is most memorably expressed in *The Second Discourse*. Rousseau laments,

> the extreme inequalities of our ways of life, the excess of idleness among some and the excess of toil among others, the over-elaborate foods of the rich, which inflame and overwhelm them with indigestion, the bad food of the poor, which they often go without altogether, so that they over-eat greedily when they have the opportunity; those late nights, excesses of all kinds, immoderate transports of every passion, fatigue, exhaustion of mind, the innumerable sorrows and anxieties that people in all classes suffer, and by which the human soul is constantly tormented: these are the fatal proofs that most of our ills are of our own making, and that we might have avoided nearly all of them if only we had adhered to the simple, unchanging and solitary way of life that nature ordained for us (Rousseau, 1984: 84-85).

One can identify three central components of Rousseau's cultural critique; ever increasing:

a) alienation,

b) misery, and,

c) artificiality.

While these aspects of Rousseau's cultural critique are interconnected, each retains individual salience.

The importance of alienation to Rousseau's work has been much discussed (Simon-Ingram, 1991; Campbell, 2012). In his mature formulation, humanity's alienation is comprehended relative to an essential 'nature' which has been irretrievably debased (Simon-Ingram, 2012). As Rousseau states in *The Second Discourse*, modernity and the civilising process saw 'nature subjected to the law' (Rousseau, 1984: 77-78). Again, there is a connection between inner 'human nature', with its valorised pure sentiment, and the 'natural world' of Rousseau's adored plants and waterfalls (Douglass, 2015). In *Reveries of a Solitary Walker* it is symbolically, *cerastium aquaticium* that Rousseau is most delighted to encounter: a rare, delicate bloom; rarely able to exist on higher ground (Rousseau, 1979: 37). Equally, Vevey, Julie's eponymous 'small village at the foot of the alps', could 'not be further from Paris' (Delaney, 2009: 28). Culture debases and alienates in a manner the philosophes fail to grasp: they have passed so far through the denaturing alienation of modernity they can no longer see its dangers (Hulliung, 1994). Their embroilment in culture has left them unable to express, or connect with, true humanity.

> They may very well know a bourgeois from Paris or London but they will never know the human (Rousseau, 1990: 388).

Rousseau is equally explicit that the debased culture corrodes tastes in an equally alienating manner: culture strips humanity of their natural desires. Wokler puts it most efficiently, Rousseau's critique is of how, in modern culture, 'savoir springs from pouvoir' (Wokler, 2001: 10).[61] Lukacs presents a similar reading of Rousseau, the 'social institution' of culture serves to

> strip man of his human essence and that the more culture and civilisation ... take possession of him, the less able he is to be a human being (Lukacs, 1972: 136).

This alienation inexorably leads to a tragic sadness; modern culture normalises a perpetual misery (Strong, 1994). This 'constant seduction away from humanness' (Strong, 1994: 156), when consciously registered, is experienced as a truly profound melancholia. Its most superficial instantiations are of unnaturally 'excess' 'toil' (Rousseau, 1984: 84), 'inflamed bowels'

---

[61] I translate this as 'taste springs from power'.

(Rousseau, 1984: 84).[62] Ultimately, through their complicity with the norms of the dominant culture, '... the people ... purchase imaginary happiness at the price of real happiness' (Rousseau, 1984: 77-78). But for Rousseau there is something distinctly 'corrupt' (Rousseau, 1984: 79); rather than merely 'tragic' to this reality. This is a truly illusory, counterfeit existence, dominated by 'artificial faculties' (Rousseau, 1984: 81). Rousseau is most explicit, his indictment of his own readership in *The Second Discourse* leaves little to the imagination: '... your culture and your habits have been able to corrupt [you]' (Rousseau, 1984: 79). It is the false civility, the debasement of the self before the social mores, that Rousseau despises. It was the 'perfidious veil' of polite society that sharpened his pen the most keenly (Wokler, 2001: 25). Again, these indictments are not merely of a polity that is unjust, or of its norms or leaders lacking legitimacy. Rousseau's cultural critique is a crucial component of his broader articulation of the obstacles to social subjects attaining the good life; the pathologies of the social.

The Pathological Colonisation of one Social Sphere by the Logic of Another

A third pertinent framing of social pathology that can be found across Rousseau's work is his diagnosis of the colonisation of social spheres by the rationalities of other social domains. Neuhouser (2012) identifies such a species of social pathology in Rousseau's *Discourse on Political Economy*. For Neuhouser it is not merely the entry into a particular social sphere of an unsuitable, damaging logic; it is the total domination of said sphere by the rationality of a distinctly alternate social dimension. By way of example, Neuhouser points to Rousseau's discussion of Marius' hiring of mercenaries to quash dissent during the collapse of the Roman Empire (Neuhouser, 2012: 634). The legions were previously bound by codes of honour, proud of their traditions and status. Introducing mercenaries was to force the logics of exchange into this social sphere. As Neuhouser comments,

> It would be unwise to saddle Rousseau with the implausible view that it is a bad thing for social relations of any kind to be mediated by money. The more plausible claim is that *certain kinds of social relations are necessarily distorted once money comes to serve as their organizing principle*. One of Rousseau's complaints here is that individuals who carry out the duties of citizens only because they are paid to do so are easily manipulated by those in power in ways that violate the appropriate ends of political life (Neuhouser, 2012: 634 – my italics).

Again, I consider Neuhouser's (2012) analysis of useful in drawing out this distinct species of social pathology. Extending beyond Neuhouser's analysis, one can readily see how such a species of social pathology is not merely located in *Discourse on Political Economy*. For instance, one can

---

[62] Recall, there is a similar discussion of the unwell polity in *The Republic,* during Socrates' discussion of the City of Pigs. Again, the problem is the deviation from the pastoral way of life, and a move towards consuming excess alcohol and fatty sauces (Plato, 2008: 373a).

read Rousseau's *On The Origins of Language* as submitting that a foundational colonisation of the communicative sphere has occurred by the dominance of exchange logics:[63]

> Whereas the words *aimez-moi* must in the past have been superseded by *aidez-moi*, now all that we say to each other is *donnez de l'argent* (Rousseau, 1997c: 298-9).

Again, this species of critique seems most appositely framed in the language of pathology. The colonisation of the communicative realm by an instrumental rationality is not, in itself, an injustice (Neuhouser, 2012: 634). Neither is the introduction of capital into the running of the armed forces an 'unjust' development. Rather, it represents a foundational harm to the social body, a challenge and threat to social functioning; and thus an impediment to social subjects attaining the good life. Viewing Rousseau's critique through this optic only serves to accentuate the limitations of the 'liberal' framing of 'justice'; and the need to engage with Rousseau as a pathology diagnostician becomes ever more salient (Neuhouser, 2012: 629). In agreement with Neuhouser (2012), I argue that this species of Rousseau's submissions, his analyses of colonising social logics, is best framed as social pathology diagnoses. I draw out the true import of reclaiming this species of social pathology in my following section.

Pathological Relations of Unstructured Dependency

Scholarly orthodoxy has long been to view Rousseau's analysis of pathologically unstructured dependency as central to his critique (James, 2013; Rousseliere, 2016). As Rousseau elaborates in the fictive anthropology of the *Second Discourse,* natural man is

> ...the most advantageously organized of all. ... [Capable of] ... satisfying his hunger under an oak, quenching his thirst at the first stream, finding his bed under the same tree, which provided the meal; and behold, his needs are furnished (Rousseau, 1984: 81).

He is thus,

> ... [a] ... free being whose heart is at peace and whose body is healthy (Rousseau, 1984: 97).

In contrast, modernity subjected man 'to universal dependence' (Rousseau, 1984: 98). Of the many harmful 'passions and caprices' of civilisation, this is perhaps the most damaging: man is most 'weak when he is dependent' (Rousseau, 1984: 83). Yet Rousseau outlines how dependence itself is a natural state (Melzer, 2006: 281). Man cannot survive without his natural needs being met: he suffers from thirst, hunger, fatigue: therefore man is naturally a dependent creature (Rousseau, 1984). It is the particularly *social* fact of modern dependency, *the unstructured nature* of man's dependence on his fellow man which is truly pathological

---

[63] This clearly presages much of Habermas' work.

(Rousseau, 1984: 125; Neuhouser, 1993: 378). While natural men 'applied themselves only to work that one person could accomplish alone'; modernity saw humanity need 'the help of another' (Rousseau, 1984: 116). It was this turn to a pathological sociality which 'first civilized men and ruined the human race' (Rousseau, 1984: 116). Today humanity is overburdened by dependence,

> ... [man] has become (a) slave ... for if he is rich he needs (the poor's) services, if he is poor he needs (the rich's) aid (Rousseau, 1984: 116).

For Rousseau, the true tragedy is that humanity has

> ... come to love domination more than independence, to wear chains for the sake of imposing chains on others in turn (Rousseau, 1984: 132).

> ... anyone must see that since the bonds of servitude are formed only through the mutual dependence of men and the reciprocal needs that unite them, it is impossible to enslave a man without first putting him in a situation where he cannot do without another man (Rousseau, 1984: 106).

There is thus an explicit complicity in humankind's continuing dependence.

It is not merely 'economic' dependency which is diagnosed in *The Second Discourse*; Rousseau is additionally at pains to articulate a state of 'moral' dependency (Dagger, 1981; Affeldt, 1999). In modernity, the human capacity to self-legislate is lost; one must submit to the power of the 'sovereign authority' which 'divine will ... [seems to] give ... a sacred and inviolable character' (Rousseau, 1984: 130). Modern subjects face a barrage of coercive obstacles which prevent them living life by virtue of their own moral judgements. Such a life precludes the possibility of attaining civic or social freedom (Dagger, 1981). It thus represents a damaging species of social pathology.

Pathologies of Recognition

There are (at least) three distinct species of recognition pathology throughout Rousseau's diagnosis (Shaver, 1989). Indeed, one might be tempted to gently echo 'Cajot's critique'[64] at this point. Read most sympathetically, these divergent framings echo Rousseau's *development* of Montaigne and Pascal in his analysis (Shaver, 1989: 261).[65] What is less controversial is that the ultimate product, Rousseau's approach to recognition-derived critique, is considerably more expansive than today's dominant 'recognition-cognitive' paradigm.

The most obvious framing of recognition pathology is of truly anthropological, macro-scale proportions: it is the 'unintended', unnatural breach of man's 'essential' monological self-

---

[64] See my earlier explanation of Cajot critique.
[65] In a fascinating paper Shaver (1989) introduces his engagement with Rousseau as a recognition theorist with quotes from Montaigne and Pascal. While Shaver does not explicitly raise Cajot's point, I think it is implicitly left hanging.

relation (Rousseau, 1984; Honneth, 2007c). As Rousseau lyrically expresses in *The Second Discourse,*

> Each began to look at others and to want to be looked at himself; he who was most handsome, the strongest, the most adroit or the most eloquent became the most highly regarded ...

> As soon as men learned to value one another, and the idea of consideration formed in their minds, everyone claimed a right to it; and it was no longer possible for anyone to be refused consideration without affront (Rousseau, 1984: 114).

In sharp contrast to the idealised self-reliant figure of Rousseau's fictional anthropology; following the breach of man's primary monological self-relation, it became impossible for humanity to truly experience contentment without attaining intersubjective recognition. People began to,

> ... attach importance to the gaze of the rest of the world, and ... (knew) how to be happy and satisfied with themselves (only) on the testimony of others, rather than on their own (Rousseau, 1984: 136).

This pathological need for recognition is a result of a foundational recognition pathology, precipitated by a merely contingent, anthropological catastrophe.

A secondary species of recognition pathology, subtly distinct from the former, is the rise of *Amour-Propre* relative to *Amour-de-soi* and *Pitie* (Rousseau, 1984). It is worth distinguishing this framing of pathology from the aforementioned. The titanic rupture of the monological self-relation is not, in itself, a cause for suffering. In a utopian social world all subjects may, potentially, be able to realise themselves through the recognition provided by others. Indeed, Rousseau's *Social Contract* aims to present a means of regulating *Amour-Propre* for the good of the republic. It is worth stressing that the conflagration of *Amour-Propre*, while a direct consequence of the breach of humanity's natural self-regard in Rousseau's narrative, does not necessarily have to develop in the manner Rousseau described. That 'natural pity ... suffered dilution' (Rousseau 1984: 132) is not an inexorable consequence of the primary breach, the foundational recognition pathology. There is a contingent basis to the current pathological recognition order. While *The Social Contract* would be unable to heal the original rupture, it seeks to ameliorate this secondary species of recognition pathology.

Thirdly, there is a framing of recognition pathology in the manner closest to its usage today, of an irrational recognition order which impedes subjects' self-realisation. People are esteemed, not for their humanity and kindness, but for their relational standing. For Shaver this directly precipitates Rousseau's critique of private property and the division of labour (Shaver, 1989: 268) The sole metric of recognition has become esteem itself. *Amour-Propre* has come to run amok. Such is the case with property as much as with people; as Emile's tutor instructs, use value has been displaced, the bourgeoisie only values that which will further its social standing: *nolo habere bona nisi quibus populus inviderit* (Rousseau, 1911: 149).[66]

A sentiment memorably expressed in Rousseau's *Letter to d'Alembert*,

> ...nothing appears good or desirable to individuals which the public has not judged to be such (Rousseau, 1960: 67).

Again, it is worth distinguishing this framing of recognition pathology from the two expressed above. This sub-set of recognition pathology does not refer to the foundational rupture of self-regard (1). Neither does it refer to the imbalance of *Amour-Propre, Amour-de-soi* and *Pitie* (2). Rather, this refers to the manner in which *Amour-Propre* is bestowed, the way in which social subjects are granted esteem. As Rousseau establishes above, it is not merely the case that *Amour-Propre* has come to dominate: it is the case that the desire for esteem can only be met by being esteemed itself. At the Palace of Fountainbleu, kindly, natural sentiment is not regarded. Rather, it is those who are esteemed by others that are respected, regardless of the content of their character, or the naturalness of their sentiments (as Rousseau would frame it).

I am not claiming to present a complete list of the multiple framings of recognition pathology that exist within Rousseau's work. Neither have I attempted to produce a complete account of the multiple framings of pathology more broadly which undergird Rousseau's rich and penetrating social critique. Rather, the purpose of this section has been to sympathetically reconstruct the most potent and pertinent framings of social pathology diagnosis in Rousseau's work.

Rousseau's framings of social pathology diagnosis *pace* the dominant recognition orthodoxy

I commenced this chapter by justifying my turn to Rousseau as an initial point of departure for the project of resurrecting the theoretical infrastructure required for a potent, critical, social pathology diagnosis. Developing from this, I drew out five distinct framings of social pathology which can be found throughout Rousseau's work which harbour the potential to challenge the dominant 'recognition-cognitive' and 'pathologies of recognition' framings. In this third and final section of this chapter, I seek to explicitly articulate how Rousseau's corpus offers today's social theorists the resources to challenge the contemporary orthodox framing of social pathology. I make three claims:

    a) Through Rousseau's analysis of pathological social dynamics (established above), he demonstrates the importance of thinking of pathologies of the social which are not

---

[66] I translate this as 'I only want a good if the people want it'.

exclusively cognitive. Rather, there exists pathologies which transcend the individual: there are pathologies of the social realm itself.

b) Drawing on from the above, Rousseau's analysis of social logics colonising distinct social spheres demonstrates how, *even when there is a cognitive aspect to social pathologies*, these maladies may be most appositely located in social processes themselves. They are thus not to be diagnosed solely 'within the head' (Freyenhagen, 2015: 136) of the individual.

c) Finally, I return to my central submission: that Rousseau's turn to a plethora of non-recognition framings of social pathology can only serve to support my critique of an exclusively recognition framing. That Rousseau, a (if not *the*) central figure in the development of recognition in social theory (Neuhouser, 2008), finds such a paradigm, without alternate theoretical resources, untenable, is deeply significant.

The Importance of Pathological Social Dynamics

It is worth stressing the true disconnect between Rousseau's critique of pathological social dynamics and today's dominant 'recognition-cognitive' lens. A targeted reading of Neuhouser's (2012) analysis can help clarify the true breadth of this distinction. While for Zurn (2011) and Honneth (2014a, 2014b), the champions of the 'recognition-cognitive' paradigm, pathologies are best grasped as 'second-order disorders' (Zurn, 2011: 345). Such disconnects operate through a

> ... [f]undamental disconnect between first-order contents and the subjects' reflexive grasp of the origins and character of those contents, where that gap systematically serves to preserve otherwise dubious social structures and practices (Zurn, 2011: 348).

Zurn is explicit that,

> ... [w]ithout the second-order disconnect, what we might generically call "bad" acts of recognition (misrecognition, non-recognition) are not ideological ... and [therefore] cannot count as social pathologies (Zurn, 2011: 349).

Rousseau's analysis sits in direct opposition to this narrow framing of social pathology, which necessitates a) a recognition framing b) a cognitive disconnect and c) such a disconnect furthers a deliberately manipulative or exploitative logic. In contrast, for Rousseau,

> [T]he feature[s] of societies that makes them susceptible to falling ill ... [are] ... the presence of social forces *that easily escape the consciousness and control of the individuals subject to them*[,] and that bring about consequences not intended by social members themselves, including the most powerful among them (Neuhouser, 2012: 637 – my italics).

For Rousseau, these social dynamics often occur when no individual intends 'pernicious consequences' or 'approves' of their ultimate outcome (Neuhouser, 2012: 637). Ultimately such pathologies are the result of 'social forces' *beyond the subject* (Neuhouser, 2012: 637). In total accord with Neuhouser, I argue that Rousseau's diagnosis is explicitly one of 'social' currents, of logics and dynamics which have gone awry, independent of human cognition, independent of human agency. These are not *necessarily* ideological dynamics, and do not *necessarily* have to further the interest of a set class of social actors. Social pathologies, in such a framing, are held to exist in a register removed from the cognition of social actors, are held to exist at an ontological level distinct from that of the cognisant subject. Such pathologies occur unmediated by human action, akin to the dynamic between the first and last terms of a geometric progression" (Rousseau, 1968: 103). These are pathologies of a different ontological strata: they are pathologies of the social itself.[67] Thus, Rousseau's framing of social pathology here sits at substantial variance to the dominant, 'recognition-cognitive' orthodoxy.

That stated, while such social ills may occur entirely disconnected from logics leading to human gain, and disconnected from any human cognition, they do not have to. While Zurn (2011) introduced, and Honneth (2014a) endorsed, tight, restrictive framings of social pathology, Rousseau's critique of pathological social dynamics is substantially more open ended. Indeed, such dynamics may function entirely to the benefit of a social class, and to the detriment of another. It may involve an explicitly cognitive aspect. Or it may not. The crucial analysis here is that Zurn and Honneth's framing damagingly excludes alternate, non-ideological, aspects of social pathology. A return to Rousseau's social-theoretical infrastructure once again makes these social maladies visible and intelligible.

Indeed, Rousseau's perspective is particularly useful because both framings may occur concurrently: the pathology may exist beyond the level of the thinking subject, but, due to the operation of ingrained social structures, may operate so as to further the material advantage of a particular class. This may be the case even where neither group explicitly intends to exploit the other. One can extract such a commentary from Neuhouser (2012):

> Under certain conditions a free market, for example, can systematically produce (and reproduce) undesirable consequences—huge inequalities, widespread poverty, the loss of social cohesion— without any of its participants foreseeing or intending them as consequences of their collective action. And, under easily imaginable circumstances, the inequality, poverty, and social dissolution produced at t1 virtually guarantee that, even when all future exchanges are uncoerced and formally just, those initial ills will only be worse at t2 (Neuhouser, 2012: 637).

---

[67] For a further example see Young (1990) *Justice and the Politics of Difference*, Chapter Three.

This is a powerful analysis. Once again, echoing Neuhouser, I submit that these pathological dynamics are located in the systems of social reproduction itself and occur at a higher level of social reproduction than that of the subject. This is not to state that the ultimate manifestation of the social pathology will not be experienced by the social subject: of course, social reality is perceived only by cognisant beings. The distinction that I am at pains to mark here is that while it is ultimately the social subject that suffers the ill effects of the pathological dynamic, this dynamic is not rooted in the subject itself. This is a crucial distinction, and a real limitation of the recognition-cognitive framework. Extending Neuhouser's earlier analysis, the cycles of crisis that Marx outlines in *Capital* are ultimately experienced by social subjects: that does not mean that the social pathology is best located in the social subject; or in the cognitive capacities of the social subject. Rather, the social pathology exists in the process of social reproduction; on a different ontological plane.

As my earlier analysis drew out, it is not merely market related dynamics which threaten society; rather there are numerous species of self-perpetuating damaging social dynamics: from the relationship between artists and audiences, or the city and the countryside. An engagement with Rousseau's work is of true utility as it serves to displace the restrictive and limiting recognition-cognitive framing of social pathology by clearly articulating how social pathologies exist substantially removed from the cognisant individual. *Pace* Zurn and Honneth, and in total accord with Neuhouser (2012), I contend that when Rousseau conducts such analysis, his scholarship can 'most convincingly be described in the language of [social] pathology' (Neuhouser, 2012: 637). Such social maladies are damagingly unintelligible to today's dominant 'recognition-cognitive' framing of social pathology.

An added nuance: the importance of Rousseau's rationality colonising pathologies

While very few of the pathological social dynamics Rousseau describes are located at the level of the subject's cognitive functioning, Rousseau's analysis of colonising rationalities adds a crucial nuance to the discussion. As repeatedly stated, the dominant 'recognition-cognitive' approach presents all social pathologies as cognitive disconnects, as errors in the subject's cognitive functioning, which impedes their optimum engagement within the recognition order. As established, this framing has numerous limitations (Chapter Two and Chapter Three). As discussed above, this approach locates all social pathologies 'in the head' of the social subject (Freyenhagen, 2015: 136). Rousseau's analysis of pathological social dynamics is of vital importance, in that it demonstrably locates various social pathologies as existing beyond these narrow parameters: in the social world itself.

Yet, while Rousseau's analysis of negative social dynamics serves to directly contradict the restrictive nature of the Zurn-Honnethian framing, it is Rousseau's diagnosis of rationality colonising pathologies which adds true nuance to this discussion. *Put most simply: while subjects may suffer from impeded cognitive functioning; the true origin of these pathologies must be located in the social world itself.* Thus, many cognitive pathologies are mere 'symptoms', rather than the pathologies themselves. The true pathology, as with negative social dynamics, is located in the social world and experienced by the subject, but not fundamentally of, or located in, the subject.

To further understand this subtlety, it is worth engaging with some of the subsequent framings of social pathology which utilise Rousseau's infrastructure more substantively. Of the numerous diagnoses which demonstrate a relationship between the impeded cognitive functioning of the subject and inappropriate forms of social rationality colonising the life world, it is perhaps Adorno and Horkheimer's (1997) *Dialectic of Enlightenment* that is the most renowned. For the co-authors,

> [The Enlightened] intellect … perceives the particular only as one case of the general (Adorno and Horkheimer, 1997: 84-85).

This contradiction elides with an emboldened instrumental rationality, so that

> … [M]an discards his awareness that he … is nature, all the aims for which he keeps himself alive … are nullified, and the enthronement of the means as an ends … is [irreversible] (Adorno and Horkheimer, 1997: 54).

Adorno and Horkheimer are indebted to a critique of instrumental reason which stems directly from Rousseau, via Hegel (Horkheimer, 2013).[68] The pathology central to Adorno and Horkheimer's diagnosis is of an instrumental rationality run amok; a process which, for the co-authors, has anthropological origins as ancient as the Roussean rupture of the monological self-relation. The crucial distinction here is that Adorno and Horkheimer are fundamentally presenting a totalising cognitive impediment; a failure of the subject to engage with the external world beyond the rationalities of a teleologically-driven utility calculus. This impedes both direct engagement with the social order, and equally restricts the subject's capacity for reflexivity. Yet, as with Rousseau, while the pathology is experienced, and best diagnosed through an analysis of the cognitive malfunctioning of the social subject, *the foundational pathology is not one of the subject: it is of the social*. For Adorno and Horkheimer, this is a social lifeworld where,

> … the capacity of representation is the vehicle of progress and regression (Adorno and Horkheimer, 1997: 35).

---

[68] Della Volpe (1979) has gone so far as to suggest one is best placed to read Marx directly through Rousseau, substantially displacing Hegel.

I submit that the mischief [Unwesen] preventing the reconciliation of the general and the particular is not a personal 'capacity'; a personal error: rather *a social capacity*. That, as with Rousseau's primary diagnosis, it is not a personal failure to utilise a suitable form of reason, but a social pathology. Thus, for Adorno and Horkheimer; as with Marius' introduction of capital into the legions, the form of reason is one of *social reason*. The dominant recognition-cognitive framing of social pathology lacks the theoretical resources to engage with such an understanding. Ultimately, an engagement with Rousseau's theoretical infrastructure enables the true limitations of the recognition-cognitive paradigm to be borne out. More importantly, an engagement with Rousseau presents theoretical infrastructure which can enable these domesticating lacunas to be plugged.

The Crucial Lesson from Rousseau: Recognition does not Necessitate Myopia

This engagement with Rousseau serves to destabilise the current, limited social pathology paradigm on three counts. First, as established, Rousseau, despite being the supreme recognition theorist, and having a social philosophy based around a foundational breach of recognition relations, turns to multiple framings of social pathology removed from a recognition optic. Rousseau presents, *inter alia*, pathologies of colonising rationalities, of social dynamics, of dependency, of culture, and of recognition in a much broader sense than it is utilised today. That Rousseau turns to these alternate framings of social pathology is truly telling: the most prominent classical recognition theorists does not attempt a critique of the social without alternate, non-recognition framings, to support his analysis. This serves to further illuminate the restrictive, and entirely unnecessary boundaries placed on the pathology framework as practiced by today's dominant critical social theorists. Rousseau demonstrates that it is not essential to stick rigidly to a recognition optic to analyse the pathologies of the social; *even when you are basing your entire philosophy on a foundational recognition pathology*.

Further, as established, Rousseau's scholarship underscores two additional limitations of the current framework. Firstly, social pathologies can be located in the social body itself, in processes of social reproduction. It is important to analyse social pathologies that are not located only in the subject. This is not to state that the subject cannot suffer from, or indeed be the location of, social pathologies. Rather, it is to state that only analysing social pathologies that are ultimately located within the subject, serves to artificially and damagingly restrict the social theorist's capacity to engage with the breadth of maladies existing in the social realm.

Secondly, while not all pathologies are located at the level of the subject's cognitive capacity, many are best diagnosed through an analysis of the impeded state of the social subject's rationality. There may indeed be cognitive disconnects, which are essential to the social pathologist's diagnosis. That stated, social subjects failing to grasp the reality of their environment, or utilising an inappropriate form of reason for a certain social domain, does not necessitate that the social pathology is, essentially, located within the subject's critical capacities. Rather, there may be crucial social dynamics which are only experienced, and determinable, through an analysis of the subject. That does not mean that the foundational social pathology exists in the subject. There may be foundational, anthropological bases for the sub-optimal operation of a social subject's cognitive capacity.

Rousseau's scholarship serves to underscore the importance of social pathology diagnosis. His analysis transcends the 'liberal' framings of 'justice' and 'legitimacy' (Neuhouser, 2012). Through this engagement with Rousseau's social theory, and his social theoretical infrastructure, I have outlined the import of utilising Rousseau's work to draw out the limitations of today's dominant, 'recognition-cognitive' framing of social pathology.

Conclusion

A critical engagement with Rousseau is an essential point of departure for an attempt to regain the potency of social pathology diagnosing critique, and to expose the limitations of the dominant recognition-derived frameworks. Rousseau has been presented as the social pathologist *par excellence*. While his *oeuvre* is ultimately animated by his diagnosis of a foundational recognition pathology, his analysis is never limited to a singular, restrictive, recognition optic. While the rise of an inflamed *Amour-Propre* is central to his diagnosis, Rousseau's engagement is never restricted to the subject, nor to the cognitive. As the *citoyen de Geneve's* 'protosociology' (Noone, 1980: 90) demonstrates, a critical engagement with society that seeks to 'go beyond' the questions of legitimacy and injustice (Noone, 1980: 67) necessitates a form of analysis which is not artificially restricted to the recognition order, or to the cognitive. Rather, as Rousseau's breadth, and indeed the beauty of his prose, draws out, a polycentric approach to social critique has been superior from the inception of social theory.

Chapter Five

Pathologies of Reason: Left-Hegelianism and Social Pathology

Introduction

This thesis started out by outlining the importance of social pathology diagnosing critique (Chapter One) and exposing the limitations of the dominant recognition-theoretical approach to social theory (Chapter Two). It then tracked how the contemporary study of social pathologies has come to be dominated by a limited, recognition-theoretical imagination (Chapter Three). To counter the transition to viewing social pathologies solely in this restrictive manner, I first turned to Rousseau, who I identified as the progenitor of pathology diagnosing social critique. I drew out an important irony: that while Rousseau is held today as the recognition theorist *par excellence*, he operated with a plurality of framings of social pathology unintelligible within the recognition paradigm (Chapter Four). My engagement with Rousseau started my exploration of alternate framings of social pathology which are needlessly excluded by the recognition lens (Chapters Four to Six). The objectives behind such research are twofold: a) to recover lost pathology diagnosing resources, and b) to further the case for moving beyond the restrictive recognition perspective. In keeping with these aims, this chapter presents an engagement with the various 'pathologies of reason' framings, seeking to extract the useful insights common to the competing approaches. As with the previous chapter on Rousseau, through this discussion, I seek to recover efficacious framings of social pathology which have been lost in the recognition turn.

While this thesis is strongly opposed to the dominance of an exclusionary recognition approach to engaging with the social world, it is impossible to deny the lucidity and simplicity of the recognition model (Laitinen, Särkelä and Ikäheimo, 2015). This is central to the intuitive appeal of Honneth's own Critical Theory (Anderson, 1995). Such clarity is not in abundance in the literature on pathologies of reason: this is philosophically dense material, rife with seemingly contradictory definitions and competing interpretations (Freyenhagen, 2015).[69] Further, the very meaning of the word 'reason' as utilised by Critical Theorists, is at considerable variance from its colloquial usage.[70] In contrast to the common English definition, for Hegel, Adorno, Lukacs and Honneth, *inter alia*, 'reason' is understood in a 'thick' and 'social' manner, manifest

---

[69] Honneth's *Pathologies of Reason: On the Legacy of Critical Theory* (2007b) brings together eleven previously published essays, all of which utilise a subtly distinct understanding of a pathology of reason. This text underscores how the language of 'pathology of reason' is used without specificity and more as a vague nod to a left-Hegelian legacy.

[70] I would present the colloquial understanding of reason to be something akin to the mind's capacity to understand and form judgements.

as much in forms of social organisation as in subjects' cognitive capacities (Honneth, 2007b; Strydom, 2011). For the Critical Theorist, 'reason' thus has a distinctly *social* inflection (Marcuse, 1969). To draw out this understanding in the associated literature this approach to 'reason' is often referred to as 'historically mediated reason', or 'socially mediated reason' (Marcuse, 1969; Guess, 2004; Honneth, 2007b, 2007c, 2010).[71]

Honneth has repeatedly revised his understanding of what constitutes a pathology of reason, both in his writings on the history of Critical Theory (1991, 2000, 2004a, 2007a, 2007b, 2007c, 2007d, 2010) and in his own Critical Theory of Recognition (1995, 2008, 2014b) (Freyenhagen, 2015). This has served to further complicate an already inaccessible literature (Freyenhagen, 2015: 131-132). There are thus multiple competing and contradictory understandings of what constitutes a pathology of reason in both contemporary and classical scholarship (Laitinen and Särkelä, 2019: 81). To bring some much-needed clarity, the first of this chapter's three sections is more clarificatory in nature. Section one, 'What is a pathology of reason?' reconstructs five different framings of pathologies of reason. This exercise is undertaken to explore central commonalities and to seek useful resources that can be incorporated in a revitalised pathology diagnosing endeavour. I thus engage with pathologies of reason framed within the following approaches:

(a) the left-Hegelian tradition,

(b) the pathologies of recognition framing,

(c) the dominance of instrumental rationality,

(d) the presence of socially induced category mistakes, and,

(e) Dialectic of Enlightenment style critiques.

Despite divergent philosophical convictions, I argue that a clear reconstruction of these different framings exposes two important commonalities. First, I identify a shared understanding of reason as 'thick' and 'social'; reason is held to be a fundamentally social 'process' which is capable of developing its own pathologies (Guess, 2004: 124).[72] Second, I argue that each reconstruction is centred around a primary dynamic or logic. In each case the subject internalises a form of impeded cognition, and then, through their own social action, serves to further enforce the conditions which precipitated their own cognitive impairment. Throughout this chapter I argue that recovering such an understanding is useful for revitalising social pathology scholarship.

---

[71] In an attempt to show the connection between the noumenal and the socially manifest, Delanty and Harris (2018) have connected this to the Kantian notion of 'regulative ideas of reason'.

[72] One can immediately see how this sits at variance from the understanding of reason posited by the conservative tradition, or as understood in broader society (Guess, 2004; Heywood, 2007).

The second section of this chapter, 'Critiques and Rejoinders', engages with three oft-repeated weaknesses of pathologies of reason accounts. The arguments that pathologies of reason approaches are, inevitably,

(a) woefully inaccessible, or, worse, obfuscating,

(b) unjustifiably teleological, and

(c) unjustifiably metaphysical

are sympathetically presented and responded to. Through an extended rejoinder, this section argues that a pathologies of reason approach need not be needlessly complex or committed to a totalising and acritical account of progress. By drawing on Thompson (2016), a brief discussion follows on whether a renouncement of metaphysics is either necessary or desirable.

This draws the chapter into its third and final section, 'Pathologies of Reason: beyond recognition-theory'. Having established that there are no foundational philosophical or political critiques which void the utility of a pathologies of reason approach, this final section articulates the utility of the twin characteristics presented as essential to a pathologies of reason approach. First, the importance of engaging with reason as 'thick' and 'social' is discussed: there is a need for critical theorists to contemplate reason more broadly as a meta-social process which impacts societal organisation as much as the subject's cognitive capacity. Second, I argue for the need to engage with the social dynamics that reinforce impeded individual cognition. I outline the utility of both insights, and demonstrate their displacement by, and incompatibility with, the ascendant recognition-derived orthodoxy.

What is a pathology of reason?

Much of the literature pertinent to the various pathologies of reason framings is philosophically dense and inaccessible (Schopenhauer, 1909; Santayana, 1916; Russell, 2015). For Schopenhauer (1909), this is not merely incidental, such presentation is deliberately abstruse to hide the reality that the authors have nothing of merit to say. In the 'general mystification' of Hegelian thought, Schopenhauer saw only 'pure nonsense' (Schopenhauer, 1909: 22). The fact that readers saw meaning, let alone utility, in the 'senseless and extravagant mazes of words', was, for Schopenhauer, an embarrassing 'monument to German stupidity' (Schopenhauer, 1909: 22). Yet, *pace* Schopenhauer, Critical Theorists have long identified merit in pathologies of reason approaches (Honneth, 2004a: 336-338), and, in so doing, routinely return to the foundational Hegelian insights which animate their broader project (Marcuse, 1969). For Honneth, the diagnosis of pathologies of reason is the 'explosive charge' of Critical Theory in that it connects the interdisciplinary research project with a foundation in radical left-Hegelian philosophy (Honneth, 2004a: 338). The pathologies of reason perspective can thus be understood as being both foundational for Critical Theory, but also problematically inaccessible (Guess, 2004; Honneth, 2007a, 2007b, 2007c). With such a realisation, it becomes apparent that there is an urgent need to transpose the unyielding philosophical approach into a more pliant and lucid social-theoretical register. In this exercise I grant disproportionate space to reconstructing the left-Hegelian engagement with pathologies of reason. This is because Hegelian insights recur with varying degrees of centrality in the four remaining framings. Indeed, Honneth has gone so far as to argue that,

> In all ... approaches to Critical Theory, the same Hegelian idea ... is continually incorporated, only in different characterizations of the original human practice of action (Honneth, 2007c: 25).

It is therefore unsurprising that the literature on pathologies of reason focuses overwhelmingly on the left-Hegelian approach (Marcuse, 1969; Guess, 2004; Honneth, 2007b).

I present two fundamental commonalities across the five rival framings. First, I argue that one can read an understanding of 'reason' as 'thick' and 'social' in character, existing as much in the manifest social world as in 'the head' of the social subject (Freyenhagen, 2015). In each perspective, the cognition of the agent is held to be fundamentally socially mediated. This is in direct opposition to the autonomous, atomistic agent of liberal thought, or the limited fallen agent of conservative theory (Heywood, 2007). Indeed, one can argue that all pathologies of reason approaches sit closer to Marxist or post-structuralist understandings of the relationship between the subject's cognitive capacities and broader, external dynamics. Second, I argue that in each perspective one can read a common logic: the subject internalises a form of impeded thinking, and then, through their social action, proceeds to further enforce the social conditions which, in full or in part, precipitated their own cognitive impairment.[73] Through the transposition of the abstruse philosophy into a more accessible sociological register, this reconstructive exercise seeks to disclose these two commonalities as the central insights offered by a pathologies of reason perspective.

While this chapter admits to the difficulty of the literature, *pace* Schopenhauer (1909), I do not view this complexity as synonymous with obfuscation or worthlessness. The challenge for

---

[73] For the purpose of this present project, I simply wish to outline how a dynamic exists where deficient forms of cognition are internalised (with regularity, if not total uptake) which then can lead to subjects acting in a manner which reaffirms the pathological social conditions which precipitated their impeded cognition. In this crude framing the suggested dynamic seems overly deterministic and unnuanced. In a broader project I would be keen to add further timbre to this dynamic, suggesting a more detailed account for how the subject is interpellated, to different degrees, by deficient forms of rationality by engaging with competing Althusserian, Gramscian and Giddensian framings.

my reconstructive exercise is to achieve a lucidity and clarity while retaining the philosophical richness of the left-Hegelian tradition.

Left-Hegelianism: on the pathologies of the socially mediated present

Critical Theory's engagement with pathologies of reason has clear origins in the left-Hegelian tradition (Marcuse, 1969: 7; Honneth, 2007a, 2007b, 2007c, 2014a). First generation Frankfurt School scholars produced seminal work on both Hegel and the left-Hegelian tradition more broadly (Marcuse, 1969). The origins of the left-Hegelian approach to diagnosing pathologies of reason lie across Hegel's socio-political philosophy (1970, 1991), his philosophy of history (1953) and his logic (2015). The aim of this section of the chapter is thus to explicitly draw out the left-Hegelian approach to diagnosing social pathologies, and, through doing so, to clearly articulate the fundamental steps which lie at the heart of this mode of pathology diagnosing critique.

A form of 'Reflective History' called 'Universal History' is of central importance to Hegel (Hegel, 1953; Solomon, 1970).[74] Such a discipline focuses on one meta-process, namely the inexorable unfolding of reason [*Geist*] over time. This meta-process is central to Hegelian philosophy and holds a foundational role in the left-Hegelian diagnosis of pathologies of reason (Marcuse, 1969). From the perspective of Hegel's 'Universal History', reason [*Geist*] is understood metaphysically. While *Geist* is famously hard to define (Marcuse, 1969; Solomon, 1970; Houlgate, 2012), it is perhaps best understood by Houlgate (2012) as an amalgam of the English words 'reason', 'self-understanding' and 'spirit'. For Hegel, the entirety of human culture and history can be understood as the process of abstract *Geist* finding form ('being actualised' [*Verwicklichung*]) in institutions and forms of cognition.[75] It is through overcoming ('sublating' [*Aufheben*]) the internal contradictions of the present (inadequacies in societal organisation, limited forms of thought etc) that *Geist* unfolds. In this process irrational (or pathological) forms of thought and societal organisation are displaced by more rational forms of social existence.

There is a clear eschatological nature to the Hegelian imaginary (Tucker, 1964: 45-48). In Hegelian terms, spirit continues unfolding until the 'rational universal'[76] is attained across all societal institutions (Marcuse, 1969; Honneth, 2007a, 2007c). The ultimate destination of the

---

[74] 'Universal History' is presented in contrast to 'Original History' (written by a historian living in the time depicted), or the 'Pragmatic', 'Specialized', or 'Critical' forms of 'Reflective' History. This is a particularly Hegelian demarcation, distinguishing his approach from the preceding Kantian understanding established in 'Idea for a Universal History with a Cosmopolitan Purpose' (1784, see Kant, 1996: xx).

[75] As Tucker words it, for Hegel, 'world history is thus the unfolding of Geist in time, as nature is the unfolding of Geist in space' (Tucker, 1964: 47).

[76] Where there is no lacuna between the rational potential inherent in a process and the means of its material manifestations: where society, or an aspect of society, is functioning as perfectly as it is possible for it to do so.

Hegelian social-philosophical [*Rechtsphilosophie*] project is 'reconciliation' [*Versöhnung*]: both of *Geist* with the world and of humanity with modernity (Hegel, 1991: Preface; Hardimon, 1992).[77] Marcuse argues that Hegel truly 'believed that such objective concepts and principles exist' (Marcuse, 1969: 7).[78] For left-Hegelians, the development of reason, and the diagnosis of its 'pathologies' needs to grasped relative to the 'totality' of this expansive imagination (Marcuse, 1969: 7).

From the Hegelian perspective, *Geist* is manifest in both social structures and in individual cognition; a mediating metaphysical substrate which both gives form to social life and is manifest within social life (Hegel, 1953). 'Reason' [*Geist*] is thus a mediating presence between the subject and the organised social world, which is constantly unfolding its contradictions. It is only from the position of 'Universal History' that the true development of reason can be grasped. While this remains an admittedly vast, imprecise definition, it is enough to demonstrate the core features of the Hegelian understanding. One can see how the development of individual cognition is fundamentally tied to the development of the social world, and, in particular, to the organisational rationality of social institutions. There exists a mediating process (the unfolding of *Geist*) between the individual and their capacity for optimal cognition (what would be called 'reason' to a liberal) (Hegel, 1953). It is the socially mediated reason of the present, the unfolding of *Geist*, which determines the cognition of the subject. From such a position, one can see how the subject's capacity for cognition is fundamentally mediated, and how 'reason' is understood in a 'thick' and 'social' manner.

For Hegel, 'Universal History' had (allegedly) reached its conclusion in the early nineteenth century with Junker-dominated Prussia. 'Reconciliation' [*Versöhnung*] was held to have occurred: the unfolding of spirit was complete. There were no more social pathologies in existence, as, for Hegel,

> social pathologies were to be understood as the result of the inability of society to properly express the rational potential already inherent in its institutions, practices, and everyday routines (Honneth, 2007c: 23).

However, for Hegel, within the Prussian state, the rational potential had been attained. There were thus no more social pathologies, at least not in the manner understood by Hegel. The challenge was simply for individuals to realise the rational perfection inherent in the social

---

[77] For an extended discussion, see Tucker (1964).
[78] Pippin's (1981) account is more figurative, focusing on the realm of ideas, rather than an actual moment of eschatological rupture. In this regard Pippin seems to follow Haym's canonical *Hegel Und seine Zeit*.

system: for the individual to be reconciled with the modern world (Hardimon, 1992: 165-167),[79] and to personally attain the knowledge of the contemporary unfolding of reason, or, as Hegel phrased it: to work through the *Phenomenology of Spirit*. Through reading Hegel's text, the social subject would be able to attain the perfection in their own manner of thought that was reached by the organisational structure of society. Hegel's two most famous texts, *Philosophy of Right* and *Phenomenology of Spirit* might, therefore, both be considered deeply politically conservative. For Hegel, when the reader has read (and understood) the *Phenomenology of Spirit* they will (allegedly) be able to achieve the highest possible standard of rational outlook in their own cognition. Equally, through a reading of *Philosophy of Right,* the reader will be able to comprehend the perfection of the Prussian system. There is limited, if any, need for further transition.

However, Hegel's work has long been subject to conflicting interpretations (Pippin, 1981: 509-510; Houlgate, 2012). While conservative elements utilised his texts to justify the political conjecture of the day (the so-called 'Right-Hegelians'), many progressives saw the utility of Hegel's texts in their method rather than in his conclusions (Harris, 1958). Those who utilised Hegel's approach, yet disagreed that the Prussian state was the 'reconciliation' [*Versöhnung*] of the unfolding of Reason [*Geist*] in the world [*Welt*], are referred to as 'left-Hegelians'.[80] Such figures famously included Feuerbach, Bauer, Stirner, and of course, Karl Marx. The foundational tenets of such an approach remain central to many of the pathologies of reason approaches utilised by Critical Theorists today (Honneth, .

For left-Hegelians,

> ... [t]he existence of ... such social suffering, is explicable only as the given social world exists as an 'insufficient appropriation' of an 'objectively' already possible reason (Honneth, 2007c: 23).

Thus, the development of spirit is held to be continuing: social suffering remains, therefore, *Geist* must not have completed its unfolding (Harris, 1958). With this awareness, the task then becomes to further the development of the unfolding of spirit, by engaging with, and critiquing the obstacles to, reason's development. Strydom (2008) presents this as the 'Gordian knot' which left-Hegelians seek to unpick. For a purist left-Hegelian, the challenge is to identify the pathologies of reason in the present, enabling the organisation of society to be restructured in accordance with the full force of reason. Indeed, there is a political and an ethical imperative to do so (Harris, 1958: 609). As Honneth words it,

---

[79] In my conclusion I argue that such reactionary forms of Hegelianism have come to hold an unhealthy influence on contemporary Critical Theory.

[80] They are also referred to as 'Young Hegelians', however for simplicity I stick to the term 'left-Hegelian' in this project.

> Any deviation from the ideal [non-pathological] ... must lead to a social pathology insofar as subjects are recognisably suffering from a loss of universal, communal ends (Honneth, 2007c: 24).

From such a position it becomes possible to understand the limitations of the contemporary capitalist world in purely Hegelian terms, where

> ... [the] pathological deformation by capitalism may be overcome only by initiating a process of enlightenment among those involved (Honneth, 2007c: 21).

The left-Hegelian Critical Theorist is able to provide such 'enlightenment' by diagnosing the pathologies of reason in the present, by exposing the areas of the social world where the 'rational universal' is yet to be attained and where the immanent reality of the form of social organisation falls short of the standards of 'objectively possible reason' (Hegel, 1953; Marcuse, 1969). The task is to 'practically remedy' the gulf between the organisation of the social world and the rational potential latent within it (Honneth, 2007c: 21). In Marcuse's words,

> As long as there is any gap between real and potential, the former must be acted upon and changed until it is brought into line with reason (Marcuse, 1969: 11).

Such pathologies in the development of reason can exist in any social domain: in the organisation of sexual relations, in the modes of economic exchange, or in the forms of aesthetic appreciation (Hegel, 1953: Part Three: Section C; Honneth, 2007c: 23-27). Thus, the challenge is to subject society as a 'totality' to continual, rigorous critique (Honneth, 2007c: 24).[81] [82] For example, for Honneth (2007c), Marx's critique of the irrationality of the capitalist system can be read as deeply left-Hegelian, that is as a diagnosis of a pathology in the dominant form of reason. Transposed into the left-Hegelian register, Marx's critique of the capitalist economic system can be understood as the argument that the current form of economic organisation is inferior to the potential for a more rational form of exchange which is practically attainable (Honneth, 2007c: 24). Similarly, Honneth reads Freud's critique of the inadequacies of the repressive form of sexual relations can be comprehended as an argument that the current, immanent practices of expressing sexuality were inferior to the potential for a more rational form of sexual life, which had already been made possible by the unfolding of *Geist* (Honneth, 2007c: 24-26). Returning to Honneth's explanation:

> In all ... approaches to Critical Theory, the same Hegelian idea – namely, that a rational universal is always required for the possibility of fulfilled self-realization within society – is continually incorporated, only in different characterizations of the original human practice of action (Honneth, 2007c: 25).

Within the left-Hegelian approach to diagnosing pathologies of reason, the potential for transcendence is implicit in the critique of the contradictions immanent to the lifeworld

---

[81] Hegel frames this as the need to look all the 'negatives in the face' (Hegel, 1970: 36).
[82] For Freyenhagen (2013), Adorno's radical negativism in *Negative Dialectics* (1966) retains a sensitivity to the centrality of negation, and of negativity, in Hegel's dialectical method.

(Strydom, 2011). It is with reference to the diagnosis of social pathologies of reason that Critical Theorists developed their distinctive framing of 'immanent-transcendence'. For Hegel, it was essential that the theorist sought to 'penetrate into the immanent content of the matter' (Hegel, 1970: 52), to explore the latent potentialities (the more sophisticated forms of reason) within the present. Diagnosing pathologies of reason presents opportunities for 'immanent-transcendence' (Strydom, 1989). Through an analysis of the latent potentialities for a more rational society that exist within the present, the possibilities of a more rational future can be articulated (Strydom, 1989: 2). From such a perspective the potential for transcendence of the given lies dormant within the immanent lifeworld, which can be attained by the 'sublation' [*Aufheben*] of the contradictions of the lifeworld.

The final component of the left-Hegelian approach to diagnosing pathologies of reason that needs to be explicated is the relationship between the individual subject and the broader social totality.[83] How precisely does the individual's journey through the Phenomenology of Spirit connect with the Philosophy of Right, considering the central mediating and connecting role of Geist? How does the social actor fit into this grand Hegelian paradigm (Hardimon, 1992)? I argue that one can understand the relationship between the individual and the social as expressing a particular dynamic, and that this particular logic occurs, in varying manifestations across all the pathologies of reason approaches.

For the left-Hegelian, individual cognition is mediated by Geist. When the subject engages with the wider world, their cognitive capacities reflect both their own socialisation (within the society: a society which has reached a certain development of rationality) and presents the development of their own reason/self-consciousness (as expressed in the stages of the Phenomenology). The actions of the social subject thus proceed to further the form of reason which they, and the social world, have attained. Both of which are fundamentally mediated by the unfolding of *Geist*. Ultimately, one sees a *dynamic of mutual reinforcement*: where both the social organisation and the self-consciousness of the subject serve to mutually reinforce obstacles to spirit's unfolding. The diagnosis of a social pathology of reason is thus doubly 'social': the cognitive impairment in the subject is derived from a 'thick' 'social' understanding of reason. This can be presented as a negative reading of the *Doppelstatz*: if what is rational is socially determined, and what is socially determined is predicated upon the unfolding of reason (Bristow, 2014), this must also account for the presence of social pathologies of reason.[84] The

---

[83] As acknowledged above, this is a problem of real complexity which requires a more extended analysis. See Pippin (1981), Taylor (1989) and Wood (1990).
[84] Tentative nods in this direction in Honneth (2010).

subject themselves, through their engagement with the social world, with their impeded cognitive capacity, serves to reassert, or reaffirm, certain pathological irrationalities.

Despite there being substantial divergences across the various framings of pathologies of reason, this foundational logic is consistently central. To restate the dynamic: the limitations in the cognition of the individual actor are produced by their socialisation; similarly, when the actor engages with their social world, they serve to reinforce the pathologies of reason which they, themselves imbibed from the social totality.

Pathologies of recognition as pathologies of reason

The dominant recognition-derived approach for furthering social theory has a clear origin in Hegelian philosophy (Honneth, 1995; Chapter One). This heritage is particularly salient in the work of the Jyväskylä School (Laitinen, Särkelä and Ikäheimo, 2015). From such a perspective, the social world is presented as a 'recognition order', in which the fundamental subjecthood of social actors is acknowledged ('recognised') according to irrational socially determined criteria. In this way, Honneth's Critical Theory of Recognition serves to 'sociologise' Hegel's parable of the struggle for recognition of the 'unhappy consciousness' in the *Phenomenology of Spirit* (Anderson, 1995). The social world is held to be pathological if it fails to offer recognition networks commensurate with the highest level of reason attained by the social body.[85]

In Honneth's (1995) *Struggle for Recognition*, the importance of recognition relations that provide love, esteem, and respect is underscored. Such requirements are presented as foundational for the social subject to enjoy a healthy relation to self.[86] Fundamentally, by virtue of their membership of the human race, all subjects deserve to be treated with love, esteem, and recognition.[87] As the pathologies of recognition paradigm makes clear, due to pathological recognition relationships, not all social subjects are granted access to these three foundational requirements. Be it due to racial, gendered, or class dynamics *inter alia*, or to intersections between them, various social actors find themselves disadvantaged by the exclusionary nature of the recognition order. Where the recognition order fails to provide these essential facets of recognition to social subjects, the recognition theorist speaks of a 'pathology of recognition'.[88]

---

[85] While I argue throughout this thesis that the Honnethian recognition paradigm is an inadequate incarnation of the left-Hegelian tradition (Chapter Two), in this chapter my objective is merely to chart the centrality of the two central logics outlined above as central to the rival pathologies of reason framings.

[86] Honneth here extends the Hegelian reflections on the conditions for ethical life [*Sittlichkeit*].

[87] Having presented an ethical framing, this analysis proceeds to introduce a more Kantian morality [*Moralitat*] to the discussion. Honneth (2007d) expands upon his rationale in an article in *Critical Horizons*, 'The irreducibility of Progress: Kant's Account of the relationship between Morality and History'.

[88] This is expressed in greater detail in Chapter One.

Transposing this approach into the discourse of its latent Hegelianism, one can view the recognition order as expressing varying degrees of rationality (Ingram, 2010). As with the left-Hegelian framing more broadly, the recognition theorist seeks to locate the means for transition and transcendence within the immanent.[89] Within the social world, norms exist which insist on the equal right to 'love', 'respect', and 'esteem' of all agents (Honneth, 1995).[90] Recognition orders which exclude subjects from attaining these essential forms of recognition are held to be indicative of social pathologies of reason. The divide between the innate rational potential of the normative horizons of the social world and the failure of various recognition relationships to replicate these norms, mimics the structural divide between the capacity for reason latent within society and the structure of social relations more broadly for the left-Hegelian.

Once again, one can see how the understanding of various 'recognition orders' serves to frame 'reason' as 'social' and 'thick'. Subjects are granted, or denied, various forms of recognition on the basis of social logics and understandings. For example, as critical race theorists have argued, racism is not merely grounded in the ignorance of an atomistic individual (Du Bois, 2016). Rather, as expressed above, the pathologies of reason approach holds to an understanding of the subject as one whose cognitive capacities are fundamentally tied to the development of societal norms more broadly. Transposing racist denials of recognition to non-white people into a left-Hegelian register, one could argue that the racist's cognitive capacities are impeded by the inadequate instantiation of the already possible standards of reason which exist in normative social order (of universal equality), but which fail to be present within the racialised recognition order (where denials of respect to subjects on the basis of their race is socially sanctioned).

One can see the presence of a foundational dynamic between the social world and the social actor, which serves to mutually reinforce pathologies of reason. The social subject is socialised into a world of recognition relationships. Subject X spends their entire life observing subjects Y and Z being denied recognition, being disrespected and unloved. Unless subject X themselves, through an act of their own critical capacity, notices the disconnect between broader social normative horizons and the recognition order, it is more than likely that subject X will proceed to reinforce these norms in their interactions with subjects Y and Z. The socially precipitated cognitive impairment which subject X suffers from is then continually reinforced by X's own social action.

---

[89] I have explored the limitations of these claims in Chapter Two. As stated, in this section my objective is merely to underscore the common factors to the rival understandings of pathologies of reason in circulation.
[90] Especially Chapters One, Two and Three.

That said, as with traditional left-Hegelianism, there remains space for the resolution of these pathologies. According to Honnethian recognition theorists, through an exploration of subjects' experiences of disrespect and of denied recognition, immanent-transcendent critique remains possible. By examining the occasions where recognition-relationships are not developed to support love, rights and esteem (where there are pathologies of recognition), one can determine a disconnect within the immanent lifeworld. The theorist can identity an immanent contradiction between the broader social norms for equal recognition (the conditions of Ethical Life [*Sittlichkeit*], and the pathological recognition relationships which inhibit healthy recognition. Through a rigorous immanent critique of said contradictory recognition relationships, recognition theorists seek to push towards a more rational lifeworld.[91]

However, as this thesis argues, the pathologies of recognition approach is deeply problematic (Chapter Two, Chapter Three). While recognition approaches can harbour utility, for Honneth a recognition perspective *alone* is able to capture the totality of the pathologies of the social (Fraser and Honneth, 2001). There is thus no space for alternate modes of engagement (Chapter Three). As expressed, numerous forms of social pathology are hidden from the recognition lens (Chapter Two, Chapter Four, Chapter Six). Various philosophical critiques have been levelled against the paradigm's capacity to adequately engage with the complexity of power relationships which extend far beyond recognition (Chapter Two). Further, recent developments have seen the recognition approach increasingly tied to a restrictive cognitivism (Chapter Three). Thus, the radical potential of diagnosing pathologies of reason through a recognition-derived approach, as part of a more 'polycentric' and 'multilateral' Critical Theory has been lost (Fraser and Honneth, 2001: 209). My final chapter (Chapter Seven) seeks to recover this potentiality.

As this reconstructive exercise has brought out, viewing pathologies of recognition as pathologies of reason has an innate appeal (Ingram, 2010). Once again, one can see how this approach to pathologies of reason necessitates an understanding of reason as 'thick' and as 'social', that is as built into recognition orders which mediate subjects' interactions. And, yet again, one can see in this framing of pathologies of reason the presence of a clear logic of mutual reinforcement. The subject who suffers from a cognitive impairment (impeded reason) insofar as they have been raised to consider (e.g.) all poor people beneath contempt, will then, with their own social action, serve to reinforce the illogicality of a social world which victimises, or

---

[91] I express the profound limitations of this approach, and its 'domesticating' implications, in Chapter Seven and in the Conclusion. What is important here, however, is how the key features of the approach *attempt* to connect a thick form of reason with an immanent-transcendent approach.

does not recognise, working class subjects. The presence of this foundational social logic remains an essential social-theoretical insight to all diagnoses of pathological irrationality.

The dominance of instrumental rationality

Generations of Critical Theorists have argued that capitalism is dogged by a particular pathology of reason, the undue dominance of instrumental rationality (Held, 1980; Schecter, 2010). The hegemony of market logics across social institutions means that the social world is ruled by logics of equivalence in which the innate worth and distinctive features of subjects and entities are 'written off as literature' (Adorno and Horkheimer, 1997: 7). Only the characteristics essential to facilitating the achievement of defined 'ends' of exchange are engaged with (Lukacs, 1972). From the perspective of this pathological episteme, life, beauty, even tragedy are engaged with epistemically as exchangeable 'dead matter - a heap of things' (Horkheimer, 1993: 81). Such a perspective strips social action of its essential humanity: concerns of identity and individuality are entirely negated (Fromm, 1963; Horkheimer, 1993; Adorno and Horkheimer, 1997). Today, the social subject is acculturated within a world dominated by such transactional, instrumental logics (Adorno, 1978; Bronner, 2011). Adorno's (1978) *Minima Moralia* sought to expose the minutiae of this process through a series of vignettes. Children are taught from infancy how to survive in an instrumental world: act instrumentally. They must achieve the salient targets at schools, and then play the REF at university. Rationality has become synonymous for 'efficiency'[92] of productive labour. For Han (2012), there is thus a damaging loss of the potential for an 'erotic' engagement with the lifeworld: the social subject is unable to experience mimetic-erotic forms of rationality as there is an ever-decreasing space for alternate forms of social action.

The subject who has been raised in a lifeworld riven by instrumentality will likely engage with the social realm in an instrumental manner (Adorno, 1978; Horkheimer, 2014). Their socialisation leaves them ill-equipped to comprehend the *hic et nunc*, the particular, the mimetic. More damagingly, in a neoliberal social order, if a child is raised to truly appreciate alternate forms of reason, they will be unable to function in the lifeworld (Ratner, 2019). Imagine a ten-year old who fails to accept that land can be owned, or who refuses to accept that one can exchange capital for meat or for labour. Sadly, such a child would be unable to function in today's society; and, ironically, the child would be held to be subject to a personal pathology (Fromm,

---

[92] This connects to Beck's analysis of how such 'rationalisation' (in terms of streamlining and instrumentalising) in risk society has led to a new 'rationalisation' (in terms of the need for new justifications and explanations for social action, where they are increasingly disconnected from basic human needs and desires) (Beck, 1997: 16).

1963, 2010). Following Fromm, it seems essential to be able to speak of an 'insane', 'pathological' social order: crucially it is the society, rather than the child, which suffers from the pathology (Fromm, 1963, 2010).

The dominance of instrumental rationality, akin to the other species of social pathology of reason articulated, evinces a logic of reinforcement between the social subject and the broader organisation of society. The child who has been socialised to accede to the dominant normative horizon, inflected as it is with instrumental logics, will in all likelihood, through their own social action, serve to reinforce and legitimise instrumental social logics. Through engaging in capitalist exchange practices, in setting and attempting to achieve targets, in the prioritisation of certain forms of 'meaningful' social action, the subject will reinforce the dominance of the instrumental logics which precipitated their own cognitive impairment.

It is essential to stress that when subjects engage with the social world through solely (and damagingly) instrumental logics, the subject reflects the deeper social pathologies (Adorno, 1978; Fromm, 2010). As with the discussion of the left-Hegelian understanding of pathologies of reason, or the pathologies of recognition approach when transposed into the left-Hegelian register, one can see how the dominance of instrumentality is predicated on a 'thicker' understanding of reason than the liberal concept of reason as an atomistic potential dominant today. Yet again, to engage with the pathology of a dominant form of rationality one must understand 'reason' to be socially manifest, to exist within, or be embodied by, social institutions as much as within the forms of cognition of social actors. An essential component of the diagnosis of instrumental rationality *qua* a pathology of reason, is the understanding of 'reason' as 'thick' and 'social'.

One can thus again see the presence of the two essential features of the pathologies of reason approach. There remains an understanding of reason which is 'thicker' and 'social', which vastly diverges from with the popular, colloquial framing of reason which understands it solely as an epistemic capacity of the autonomous atomistic subject. One can also see the centrality of the logic of mutual reinforcement: the social subject serves to reproduce the conditions which precipitated their own cognitive impairment.

Socially induced category mistakes

While the term 'category mistake' derives from Ryle's (2002) critique of Cartesian dualism, the framing has recently been developed by Critical Theorists as an appropriate signifier for a range of social pathologies including commodification, reification and dominant logics of false equivalence (O'Sullivan, 2016). Lukacs' (1972) work on reification and false equivalence is perhaps the most accessible and widely engaged with diagnosis of socially induced category mistakes.[93] For Lukacs (1972), capitalist relations require a necessarily reifying outlook. For the social actor to survive within capitalist society they must engage with the world through a lens of 'phantom objectivity' (Lukacs, 1972: 6). The capitalist 'form of social life' (Jaeggi, 2018) necessitates a species of cognition where the social subject is unable to engage with the world in a manner compatible with the correct identification of external subjects and objects (Adorno, 1978). For first generation Critical Theorists, this represented a clear social pathology of reason (Honneth, 2000).

As Marx (1976) expressed in his writings on the commodity form, the market order is based on logics of equivalence and exchange, rather than on use value. This produces a damaging discordance for the social subject, who is naturally aware of both the distinct ontologies existing within the social world and (according to the Marxist account of human nature) is anthropologically inclined to utilise the social world on its functional merits (Mehrotra, 1991). For a subject to survive in the capitalist market they must be able to accept that three hours of their labour time is exchangeable for four sirloin steaks, or thirty-six pounds sterling. They must further be able to accept that those four sirloin steaks, at point of sale, possess an equivalent value (a shared equivalent worth) to any other commodity of equivalent market price. This foundational market logic is entirely at variance with the knowledge of the distinct ontological categories of the lifeworld. Ultimately, as Lukacs states, the necessity to obviate our understanding of the ontological distinctiveness of the constituents of the world leads to 'the reification of all human relations' (Lukacs, 1972: 6); to the 'fragmentation of the object of production' and, ultimately, to the 'fragmentation of … the subject' (Lukacs, 1972: 89). Thus, implicit within Lukacs' work is the warning that when the subject loses the ability to distinguish between ontologically distinct entities, they risk losing their own coherent relation to self (Lukacs, 1972).

Schecter draws out how such reification is not just an individual failure of cognition, but a social pathology. It must be understood as

> … an epistemological problem which can no longer be solved philosophically … [I]t is … an absolutely fundamental problem about knowledge which *requires a practical political solution* because the moment for its theoretical resolution as a knowledge problem has been made redundant by history (Schecter, 2010: 51 – my italics).

As Schecter stresses, social processes precipitate this 'fundamental problem about knowledge' (Schecter, 2010: 51). Critical Theorists thus argue that the cognitive capacities of the subject must be understood as being crucially impacted by logics which exist beyond the subject's

---

[93] It should be noted that Lukacs himself does not utilise the terminology of 'socially induced category mistakes'.

consciousness. There is a form of reason which exists, or is supported by, market logics (reifying, commodifying, equivalence based). As Schecter argues, it is not possible to provide a solution to these forms of irrationality simply through a correction of the 'knowledge problem' they represent (Schecter, 2010: 51). Rather, it is essential to understand such reificatory logics as requiring a 'practical political solution' (Schecter, 2010: 51). To cure socially induced category mistakes, the solution is to change the forms of reason which are embodied by the logics of the social world. Reason, thus, once again, is understood as being instantiated in processes and logics; once again a vastly more 'expansive', 'thick' and 'social' conceptualisation than that adhered to by the liberal canon.

For capitalist subjects to efficaciously navigate their social lives they must internalise the false equivalences of the market, which, in turn, necessitates a reifying outlook. The subject, having internalised these dynamics, then engages in the lifeworld reinforcing the social logics which precipitated their own cognitive impairment. We can thus see how market logics induce category mistakes (social subjects need to engage in calculations predicated on false equivalences). The social actor then reaffirms the irrational social world through their engagement with irrational social processes, that is, by engaging in transactions which are predicated on an ontologically reductive logic of false equivalence.

Civilisational critiques

The final approach to engaging with pathologies of reason presents as something of a return to coda. There is a clear 'World-Historical' inflection to the diagnoses of Adorno and Horkheimer. Sadly, another common feature between *Dialectic of Enlightenment* and Hegel's philosophy is their inaccessibility (Bronner, 2011). That said, as with the preceding discussion on Hegel, many contemporary Critical Theorists still consider it to be of great merit to engaging with their text: Bronner considers that *Dialectic of Enlightenment* is 'perhaps *the* great critical encounter with modernity undertaken from the left' (Bronner, 2011: 51 – my italics).

Similarly to Hegel, Adorno and Horkheimer present their work relative to a universal historical time: from 'Homeric myth' (Adorno and Horkheimer, 1997: 55) to the Culture Industry. While Hegel presents the driving force of history to be the unfolding of *Geist*, for the co-authors of *Dialectic of Enlightenment* the propulsive force of history is 'Enlightenment'. Adorno is a philosopher of extreme negativity (Freyenhagen, 2013),[94] and it is unsurprising that his

---

[94] For instance, the co-authors write that the 'curse of irresistible progress is irresistible regression' (Adorno and Horkheimer, 1997: 36).

characterisation of 'enlightenment' is deeply pessimistic. For Adorno and Horkheimer, 'Enlightenment' is understood as the process through which the 'mythic mode of apprehension' (Adorno and Horkheimer, 1997: 6) is displaced by subsumptive rationalities. A direct result of this is that the living, the affective, and the qualitative become redundant, so that the world is reduced to 'dead matter – a heap of things' (Horkheimer, 1993: 81). An essential part of this process of Enlightenment, and core to its pathological nature, is that humanity starts to locate itself outside of nature:

> ... [a]s soon as man discards his awareness that he ... is nature, all the aims for which he keeps himself alive ... are nullified, and the enthronement of the means as an end ... is already perceptible in the prehistory of subjectivity (Adorno and Horkheimer, 1997: 54).

For Adorno and Horkheimer the move to 'Enlightened' thought is deeply pathological. It is not just a pathology of reason, it is *the* overdetermining pathology of reason. What is distinctive about Adorno and Horkheimer's imagination, relative to other contemporaneous theorists, is that their pathology of reason is no modern phenomena, rather it can be traced back into the depths of human pre-history (Adorno and Horkheimer, 1997: 43-45). There is an entire excurses of the text dedicated to the argument that it is possible to 'recognize enlightened thought even in the most distant past' (Adorno and Horkheimer, 1997: 45) In their rendition of the myth of Odysseus, one can see enlightened thought existing through the relation between 'naked power', 'subjectivity' and alienation (Adorno and Horkheimer, 1997: 45-47). Humanity is already seen to be isolating itself from the *hic et nunc,* from the biological species, in its self-created fictive prehistory. For the co-authors this pathology of reason exists as much in Weberian capitalist bureaucracies as in the Homeric myths:

> ... [t]he irrationalism of totalitarian capitalism, whose way of satisfying needs has an objectified form determined by domination which makes the satisfaction of needs impossible and tends toward the extermination of mankind, has its prototype *in the hero who escapes from sacrifice by sacrificing himself* (Adorno and Horkheimer, 1997: 55 – my italics).

For the co-authors, the ascent of subsumptive rationalities is typified by Odysseus, 'the self who always restrains himself and forgets his life' (Adorno and Horkheimer, 1997: 55). The epic hero suffers from a living alienation; a prototypical petrified subject. Odysseus is tied to the mast of history, unable to embrace 'instinct' (Adorno and Horkheimer, 1997: 69), to return once again to the immediacy of existence. What further follows from the pathology of enlightened reason is the 'elimination of qualities' from the subject's perception, viewed solely as their 'conversion into functions' (Adorno and Horkheimer, 1997: 36). Before long, the capacity for a holistic, mimetic or erotic encounter with the present is 'written off as literature' (Adorno and Horkheimer, 1997: 7), incommensurate with the dictates of subsumptive rationalities. One can thus read *Dialectic of Enlightenment* as presenting a foundational pathology of reason: a direct critique on Enlightened thought as unduly subsumptive and incapable of furthering true happiness.

There is a particular form of Enlightened cognition, *the conceptual domination of the particular*, which epitomises the violence of Enlightenment thought. The pathology is where the subject engages with the lifeworld through a conceptual form of cognition to such an extent that the 'thing in itself' is negated. In the co-author's turn of phrase, the conceptual 'liquidates' the particular (Adorno and Horkheimer, 1997: 17). This foundational pathology of reason is endemic to Enlightened cognition; there is a fundamental 'incongruence of concept and actuality' (Adorno and Horkheimer, 1997: 30). As the Enlightened 'intellect … perceive[s] the particular only as one case of the general' (Adorno and Horkheimer, 1997: 84-5), it opens the possibility to engaging with the individual solely in the abstract.[95]

In a very similar way to the Hegelian imaginary, for Adorno and Horkheimer 'reason' is understood as both 'thick' and 'social' in character, it is found in the very recesses of subjectivity, in the forms of engagement with the social, and in the mode of communion with the aesthetic. Equally, the pathological forms of rationality invade the physical architecture of the present, in the way a door is closed, or the layout of chairs to desks in an office (Adorno, 1978). Indeed, the spread of subsumptive reason was held to be so pervasive for Adorno and Horkheimer that it posed methodological challenges for their critique (Honneth, 2000). The anthropological narrative, and obscure manner of presentation aside, it remains clear that Adorno and Horkheimer view 'reason' as more than just a cognitive process. Rather, 'reason' is held to be a social process, mediating the individual and the world. The pathologies of Enlightened rationality, epitomised by the conceptual domination of the particular, are thus almost impossible to avoid.[96]

Finally, it is worth reasserting the relationship between the individual and the social recurring throughout all these framings of pathological reason. Because reason is framed as more than just the cognitive capacities of the individual and is held to be manifest in forms of social life and organisation, the individual's social action perpetuates pathological irrationalities. The subject is socialised to accept and perpetuate Enlightened forms of cognition to the detriment of their capacity to engage with the world, and express an unalienated humanity. As Adorno wrote in *Minima Moralia*, 'happiness [itself] is obsolete' (Adorno, 1978: 217).

---

[95] Roberts expresses this well when he argues that Enlightened cognition (as understood by Adorno and Horkheimer) 'enables conceptuality to dispense with individuality in favor of the ability to perform a *function*' (Roberts, 2004: 63 – my italics).

[96] For Adorno, context-transcending art was perhaps the sole remaining possibility. To this end he developed a passionate interest in the atonal music of Alan Berg (Held, 1980).

Concluding thoughts on this reconstructive exercise

This reconstructive exercise drew out two features common across the five rival framings. I presented a common understanding of 'reason' as 'thick' and 'social' in character, which sits in clear contrast to the colloquial, broadly liberal, understanding. This awareness that the form of reason dominant in the lifeworld may itself be pathological is an important social-theoretical insight. Second, I drew out a shared dynamic of mutual reinforcement between the subject and the social world common to each understanding. Having been socialised with a cognitive impairment, the social subject then proceeds to act in the lifeworld in a manner that reinforces the conditions which precipitated their impeded cognition.

The limitations of a pathologies of reason approach: critiques and rejoinders

This section of the chapter sympathetically presents three of the most prominent critiques of the pathologies of reason approach.

a) That a pathologies of reason approach is inevitably mired in complexity and inaccessibility (and is thus exclusionary),

b) is necessarily based on an unreflexive and politically problematic understanding of both 'reason' and 'progress',

c) and that such approaches necessitate a problematic commitment to a form of metaphysics.

Having outlined these common (and reasonable) fears, I offer rejoinders. The purpose of this exercise is to confirm that there is no irremediable weakness to a pathologies of reason approach, before I chart the problematic exclusion of the perspective's insights from the 'recognition-cognitive' and 'pathologies of recognition' framings.

The critique of inaccessibility and obfuscation

It is routinely stated that the pathologies of reason approach, particularly in its Hegelian and Adornian manifestations, is particularly impenetrable (Bronner, 2011). It is often pointed out that the literature is overburdened by philosophical complexity, made worse by the fact that there are various terms which have multiple, and at times, contradictory meanings (Popper, 1945). One can draw a thread from Schopenhauer's acerbic caricature, through Santayana's *Egotism in German Philosophy* (1916), through the logical positivists, through Bertrand Russell's *A History of Western Philosophy* (1945), to Karl Popper's *The Open Society and its Enemies*

(1945). Philosophers and theorists from otherwise divergent schools of thought have united to condemn the pathologies of reason approach as primarily obfuscation and not worth engaging with. Fundamentally, the pathologies of reason approach is held to be irreconcilable with the requirements of lucid, accessible social theory.

There is a second aspect to this critique which builds upon the first submission of obfuscation: the work is inaccessible. If the aim of Critical Theory is to provide radical change, of actual social praxis, how can this be pursued with theoretical resources which are incommunicable to the wider social world? To these entirely reasonable and recurring critiques, I offer three responses.

It should be noted that often the Critical Theorists' unorthodox style is not merely down to a laissez-faire attitude to the clarity of their argumentation, rather the author may desire the reader to engage with their text beyond the conventional analytical register (Honneth, 2000). Often, the work is in a deliberately 'obscure manner of presentation' (Habermas, 1982: 14): think of *Dialectic of Enlightenment* or *Minima Moralia*. These are not texts to reduce to numbered theses with varying sub-arguments.[97] Diagnoses of pathological irrationality deliberately do not explicitly draw out 'causal links', or, such links are simply 'absent' (Herf, 2012: 86). Texts that present a critique of the dominant form of reason face a logical conundrum. If the hegemonic forms of understanding are damaged by colonising logics or foundational flaws, how can such a critique be expressed? Communication and cognition sit in such close proximity. Honneth (2000) suggests that Critical Theorists have sought a means out of this dilemma through 'Disclosing Critique'. Instead of utilising the dominant mores of exchange and presentation, and thereby being limited by exactly the flaws in reasoning the authors' seek to illuminate, Critical Theorists have sought to diagnose pathologies of reason more obliquely, through appeals to literature, to sensation, or through exaggeration and allegory (Honneth, 2000).[98] For Honneth (2000), *Dialectic of Enlightenment* represents an ideal-typical work of 'world disclosing' critique. For van den Brink (1997), there are crucially important components to this work which must be appreciated as both linguistic and philosophical devices. One can thus argue that exaggeration and excurses are utilised to draw out the pathologies of reason without falling victim to the same perversions of reason the authors seek to critique.

This is not to state that clarity is abound, or that such texts are effortlessly approachable. Indeed, one must admit that aspects of the pathologies of reason literature are simply poorly

---

[97] To do so would be akin to presenting Tchaikovsky's Sixth Symphony in Wave lengths and frequencies rather than as music. As Hegelian scholars, Adorno and Horkheimer would be well aware of the dangers of seeking to disconnect content from form.

[98] One can detect further contemporary resonances of this strategy in Sloterdijk's (2012) consciously 'hyperbolic' *The Art of Philosophy*.

written, and unduly complicated (Schopenhauer, 1909). As commented above, the pathologies of reason approaches do not hold the intuitive appeal of Honneth's Critical Theory of recognition. Much of the literature is complicated, unwieldy, and hard to engage with. Further, the very idea of reason as 'thick' and 'social' is difficult to connect with: it sits so far away from the mainstream understanding. However, as I have stressed previously, just because a text is inaccessible, or at odds with broader dominant mores, does not of itself mean that it is not of considerable merit. The challenge becomes to draw out the essential components of the pathologies of reason approach and to present them in a more accessible register. This has been a central objective of the preceding section of the chapter.

Finally, the question must be raised as to how a work may present itself as a 'powerful manifesto' (Roberts, 2004: 72) for liberating people from oppressive conditions when the people the text desires to liberate are unable to comprehend it. At the very least, this presents methodological questions surrounding the critical distance of the theorist to the immanent lifeworld (Honneth, 2000; Celikates, 2018). In response, I would argue that pathologies of reason approaches retain a clear connection to the immanent conditions of the lifeworld through the methodological centrality of immanent-transcendence.

Predicated on compromising teleological and universalist understandings of reason

With the rise of postmodernism, and, more recently, of decolonial and post-colonial scholarship, the idea that the theorist can identify a singular form of reason unfolding over time has been increasingly contested (Lyotard, 1984; Allen, 2016). These represent two distinct critiques, united in their scepticism that history can be charted as the development of the singular unfolding of reason. This seems particularly damaging: the explicitly Hegelian form of pathology diagnosis is wedded to an undeniably universalistic narrative. Further, in Hegel's texts, it is not merely one universal logic which effects human cognition and human society; it is the same logic which impacts nature. Recall that for Hegel nature is the unfolding of *Geist* in space. For postmodernists, critical of universal grand narratives, the idea that a singular process can be identified in the unfolding of human life is both highly doubtful and politically suspect (Lyotard, 1984). The idea that the same process can be charted to be determining the development of the natural world additionally, risks appearing simply self-parodic. Further, for post-colonialists and de-colonialists there is a deep suspicion of 'Enlightenment narratives' (Allen, 2016). For Allen, in her recent, and highly influential, *The End of Progress* (2016), Enlightenment logics are held to be inseparable from the imposition of Western, colonial knowledge systems, and have been utilised repeatedly to discredit and supplant local knowledges.

These are serious critiques and require thoroughgoing rejoinders. Indeed, if the diagnosis of pathologies of reason is fundamentally, and irremediably, a tool for colonial domination, perhaps it is simply best forgotten. Further, if the framework is inextricably tied to a singular notion of reason, unfolding universally, without located spatiotemporal distinctions, again, perhaps it is irreconcilable with the insights of contemporary decolonial, postcolonial and critical race theories. In response to these challenges, I raise three rejoinders.

First, in response to the challenge that the pathology of reason approach adheres to a dangerous and unjustifiable universalism, one can argue that while such a universal outlook was undeniably present in the initial Hegelian framework, it has been substantially obviated in its later reincarnations. The theoretical infrastructure is not static; it has evolved in response to broader progressive scholarship. For example, the diagnosis of pathologies of reason *qua* the diagnosis of reifying logics, or of instrumental rationalities, can be engaged with without any such grand universalising notions.

In response to post-colonial or decolonial challenges, one might add that engaging with such realities *qua* social pathologies may add a further theoretical lens to the arsenal of theorists seeking to engage with the petrifying and objectifying dynamics of racial hierarchies. This response is then both an acknowledgement and a modification: true, in its purest reading, Hegel presents universalist arguments.[99] However, this does not mean that such arguments are irredeemable: one can simply jettison the universalising aspects of Hegelian philosophy and retain the insightful theoretical apparatus. Or, put differently, just because the original Hegelian framing had universalist components does not mean that the apparatus presented more broadly is irredeemably connected to universalist assumptions.

Second, several responses can be raised to the challenge that the diagnosis of social 'irrationalities', or the desire to further 'Enlightened' thought, is fundamentally inseparable from racialising and colonial logics (Allen, 2017). There has long been an investment in Marxist and explicitly left-Hegelian themes in post-colonial and critical race theoretical texts (Said, 1978; Chibber, 2013). But more importantly, one could simply reject Allen's contention: an investment in the notion of progress, *does not in itself*, necessitate a colonial mindset. The roots of the Critical Theoretical project in left-Hegelianism are not irretrievably colonialist. Delanty's (2009) *The Cosmopolitan Imagination*, for example, demonstrates how such insights from Critical Theory can be used to support an explicitly difference-sensitive approach to social theory. For

---

[99] There is an increasingly intense debate on the utility of 'progress' and 'universality' across the academy. See Pinker's (2018) *Enlightenment Now*. Regardless of one's take on this issue, it is certainly not uncontested: see Bell (2018), Gray (2018), and Monbiot (2018).

Delanty and Harris (2018), Critical Theory and a difference-sensitive Cosmopolitanism are neatly aligned; their foundational insights and convictions sit in harmony rather than in conflict.

Third, in response to both critiques, one can argue that the pathology of reason perspective has developed so far from the original Hegelian insights that neither criticism remains pertinent. Adornian philosophy, for instance, is explicitly aware of its 'located-ness'. Indeed, the founding premise of Frankfurt School Critical Theory is an awareness that all social theory exists within space and time, within a politically demarcated society (Horkheimer, 1975). That is perhaps its key defining feature in comparison to 'traditional' theory (Horkheimer, 1975). Thus, much 'first generation' work is at pains to address the located nature of their own diagnoses (Held, 1980). The desire to avoid specific demarcations can be read as part of a deliberate strategy of unorthodox, world-disclosing presentation (Van den Brink, 1997).

Commitment to an unjustifiable metaphysics

Another oft-cited critique of pathologies of reason approaches is that they rely upon a strong, partisan, metaphysics. As Honneth has written, this sounds very jarring to the contemporary audience, to whom nothing might sound 'more foreign' (Honneth, 2007c: 20). Since Habermas, social theory has been expunging metaphysics from its texts in favour of a move to formal pragmatics and critical hermeneutics. As Habermas expressed in *Post Metaphysical Thinking*, the reliance of the 'First Generation' on metaphysically weighty left-Hegelianism was to henceforth remain '*unambiguously* in the past' (Habermas, 2000: 12 – my italics).

To deconstruct this analysis, there are two claims at play here: a) that the pathologies of reason approach, based on a thick and social account of reason, is inescapably tied to a metaphysics, and that b) this is philosophically unjustifiable or undesirable. Both assumptions can be questioned.

First, I contend that while the pathologies of reason approach holds to a concept of reason which is 'thick' and 'social', it does not *necessarily* need to accede to any broader substantive grand metaphysical claims. While it is entirely the case that Hegel's approach is predicated on the unfolding of metaphysical Geist, this does not mean that all subsequent framings have to retain an identical Hegelian commitment to metaphysics. The (undeniable) insight that the organisation of the social world serves to further particular forms of thinking can (obviously) be productively engaged without needing to believe a singular spirit drives all nature and humanity on its predetermined unfolding. A brief survey of the literature demonstrates that this is the case, sometimes to a fault. Honneth's Freedom's Right attempts to decouple Critical Theory entirely from the metaphysics of its heritage, with reactionary results (Thompson, 2016; Bollenbeck, forthcoming). Perhaps less controversially, I submit that it is possible to redact the metaphysical understanding of Geist while arguing that normative value positions are implicit within, and reinforced by various forms of social practice, which serve important functions in the acculturation of social subjects to broader societal goals (the logic I have repeatedly drawn out).

This leads me on to my second rejoinder: it is not necessarily ideal to seek a Critical Theory which is entirely absent of metaphysical content. Indeed, Thompson's (2016) *Domestication of Critical Theory* is very clear on the merits of re-centring a critical social ontology as a pivotal component of a reinvigorated Critical Theoretical endeavour. For Thompson,

> ... an essential aspect of the neo-Idealist turn in critical theory has been its turn away from metaphysics and towards a pragmatist conception of social practice (Thompson, 2016: 179).

> By detaching itself from the ontological questions that Hegel and Marx had pursued, neo-Idealists are unable to secure a rational, universal understanding of the dynamics of a rational social order structured by truly free agents (Thompson, 2016: 180).

In keeping with Thompson's broader project, one can see how a return to a critical social ontology would be of true merit for comprehending the impact of social structures on processes of socialisation (in Thompson's terms, their 'constitutive power'). Thompson further justifies his position,

> ... we obtain rational (i.e. critical) cognition about the world only by estranging ourselves from it, not by being folded into its immediacy. Only conceptual thought can mediate the object domain, and as concept-users, the central task is to find those concepts that can mediate the world rationally (Thompson, 2016: 180).

One may thus question whether it is indeed desirable to show how one can discard the metaphysical heritage of a pathologies of reason approach. I have argued that a pathologies of reason engagement can be conducted entirely shorn of any metaphysics. Yet, following Thompson (2016), I am tempted to agree that one is able to discover 'a much more comprehensive and more critically engaged form of social critique' (Thompson, 2016: 180) with a critical metaphysics, rather than within the neo-Idealist horizons of contemporary Critical Theory.

The Displaced Utility of the Pathologies of Reason Approach

As this chapter has drawn out, despite holding to divergent philosophical premises, and utilising different theoretical registers, the pathologies of reason approaches reconstructed here all display two important commonalities.

First, there is the understanding of 'reason' as a 'thick', 'social' domain. It is worth briefly reaffirming this commonality. In the left-Hegelian imagination, reason is understood explicitly as *Geist*, as the unfolding world-spirit, which drives human history. To the recognition theorist, recognition relationships themselves represent manifestations of the various forms of reason. It is the deficiencies of such relationships that are grasped as pathologies: where the social world fails to live up to the standards of recognition that are already possible within the development of reason more broadly. With the diagnosis of dominant forms of reason, *a la* the critique of instrumental rationality, yet again 'reason' is held to be socially manifest as much as subjectively practised. With the presence of socially induced category mistakes, it is the form of life itself which is held to manifest a certain form of deformed, pathological rationality. The social subject, that performs such defective cognition is responding to and reinforcing the pathologies of reason in the broader social domain. Finally, the civilizational critiques, offered by Adorno again hold reason as a broader, macro social process. The capacity for Enlightened thought, while individually practised, is again, socially internalised and solidified in the forms of social institutions (very much akin to the Hegelian approach).

Second, I drew out the presence of a logic common to all social pathologies of reason. The pathological irrationality of the social world serves to impact the socialisation of the subject so that they internalise the pathology (for instance, an unerringly instrumental approach to life). Then, through the subject's own social action, they then serve to further the form of pathological irrationality in the social world (uncritical market logics, false equivalences etc) which precipitated their own cognitive defect. Again, it is worth reaffirming the presence of such a dynamic across the various framings. I demonstrated how, for the left-Hegelian, the social subject is socialised within a lifeworld where the development of a form of reason enables, or hinders, the social subject from furthering the development of their self-consciousness. Further, the developments of the subject's self-consciousness determines their capacity to appreciate the benefits, or limitations, of the current form of social organisation. If the organisation of the social world fails to attain the highest possible standards of rationality made possible by the unfolding of *Geist*, then inevitably the subject will fail to attain the standards of cognition (self-consciousness) otherwise open to them. Their conduct will then proceed to reinforce the limited instantiations of reason in the present, irrational social conjecture. Similarly, with the pathologies of recognition approach, the subject will be raised to consider various recognition relationships normal: they will thus be more likely to further such affirmations or or denials of recognition. Again, such a logic is clearly visible with the dominance of instrumental rationality (the subject is socialised so as to have a defective form of cognition insofar as they fail to engage with the world in non-instrumental ways, they thus proceed to engage in forms of social action which further instrumental logics). An identical logic is present with pathological category mistakes. With the Adornian, or civilizational pathology, the logic echoes the pre-stated Hegelian framework: the subject in an Enlightened society is likely to further Enlightened forms of social action.

The merits of both insights are substantial. First, the idea that 'reason' exists as a social presence beyond the merely cognitive opens up a crucial part of the social world to critique. With such an insight, the presence of pathologies within the presuppositions of social structures, and within normative horizons becomes possible. That the social world may itself present as an insufficiently rational form of life offers an exciting opportunity for a broader Critical Theoretical enterprise (Jaeggi, 2018). Further, such an insight crucially offers a foundation for a critique of the social world on grounds other than legitimacy and justice (Honneth, 2000; Jaeggi, 2018). Put more simply, the capacity to understand reason as 'thick' and 'social' furthers the capacity for radical critique.

Second, the focus on the particular logic of reinforcement of pathological irrationalities gives the Critical Theorist a particularly potent social theoretical avenue of enquiry. The utility of such an approach returns to the previous discussion on how social pathologies often evince a particular negative dynamic (Chapter Four). The theoretical infrastructure the pathologies of reason approach provides is particularly meritorious as it singularly presents a means of identifying social pathologies, while further presenting a way of understanding their perpetuation.

Both insights are totally inaccessible to the 'recognition-cognitive' paradigm. Reason, for Zurn, is purely a cognitive capacity, and, further still, it is only impeded reflexive capacities that are presented as social pathologies. Even if Zurn's approach was expanded to view reason in a social and thick manner (which would require substantial reimagining), the approach would still restrict much of the theoretical insights offered by the pathologies of reason approach insofar as it merely engages with impeded reflexive 'second-order disconnects' (Zurn, 2011; Freyenhagen, 2015).[100] Further still, as established, the recognition-cognitive approach is annexed tightly to an exclusionary recognition lens (Chapter Two, Chapter Three). Thus, the utility of the pathologies of recognition approach presented in this chapter would also fail to be incorporated, as it is solely failures of the subject to understand the emancipatory potential of recognition logics through a 'second-order disconnect' that constitutes a social pathology.

---

[100] See the extended discussion of this point offered by Chapter Three.

The idea that there may be a dynamic stemming from a problematic societal irrationality writ large across forms of social organisation and manifest in subject's cognitive processes is simply inaccessible to an approach which focuses solely on processes 'in the head' distanced entirely from processes occurring 'in the world' (Freyenhagen, 2015).

Conclusion

This chapter has argued that a pathologies of reason approach does not have to be restricted to an inaccessible philosophical lexicon. Through a detailed reconstructive exercise, five rival framings of social pathology were presented, all of which were held to share two important social theoretical insights. I have argued that the pathologies of reason approach centres an understanding of 'reason' which transcends the liberal understanding of individual cognitive capacity. Rather, to the Critical Theorist invested in diagnosing pathologies of reason, 'reason' is understood in a much 'thicker' and 'social' manner. Reason is thus understood as being embodied in forms of societal organisation as much as it is manifest in the cognition of subjects. Further, I have argued that all pathologies of reason approaches draw out the presence of an important social logic: a dynamic in which social irrationalities are internalised by actors, who, through their own social action, proceed to reaffirm the very irrational social processes which initially precipitated their cognitive impairments.

Through the sympathetic presentation of the common critiques presented against the pathologies of reason approach, and through offering measured rejoinders, this chapter has argued that the insights offered by the pathologies of reason approach are philosophically and politically justifiable. This is not to say that the various manners of diagnosing pathologies of reason are without reproach. Rather, the very real complications and complicities which are evinced (a trend towards universalism, for instance) can be distanced from the more insightful social theoretical material.

Ultimately, this chapter thus concludes in concord with the previous chapter on Rousseau: the dominant recognition-derived approaches to diagnosing social pathologies serves to needlessly exclude efficacious forms of engagement with social pathologies. There is thus an urgent need to reconsider the restrictive framing of social pathologies prevalent today so that the insights of the pathologies of reason approach, as much as the various framings of pathology presented by Rousseau (Chapter Four) and Fromm (Chapter Six), can be utilised in a broader, 'polycentric' and 'multilateral' (Fraser and Honneth, 2001: 209) Critical Theoretical endeavour.

Chapter Six

Reconstructing Erich Fromm's 'pathology of normalcy'

Introduction

This chapter argues that Erich Fromm's study of 'pathological normalcy' offers promising social-theoretical resources to help transcend the contemporary, 'domesticated', diagnosis of social pathologies. I present Fromm's framework as comprising three distinct but interconnected components:

a) an analysis of the social world as incommensurable with the demands of 'normative humanism',

b) where subjects fail to realise this due to 'socially patterned defects', and

c) where such a pathological state is reinforced as the norm through the process of 'consensual validation'.

Having distinguished these elements of the social pathology of normalcy, I show their potent aggregation in Fromm's framing of alienation.[101] In Fromm's understanding of alienation, 'the cognitive' and 'the material' are not merely united but are explicitly connected to social-structural dynamics. I explicitly draw out how Fromm's approach to social pathology can offer a palliative to the limitations of the dominant 'recognition-cognitive' and 'pathologies of recognition' approaches to social pathology scholarship.

The chapter then defends Fromm's framework[102] from the dominant criticisms which have dogged his work. Fromm presents as a thinker steeped in gendered discourse, and as entirely at odds with the ethical-cultural relativism of post-modernity (Thompson A, 2009: 43; Thompson M J, 2014; Ratner, 2014). I argue that it is both possible to substantially expiate Fromm from such charges, and that the utility of his social theoretical infrastructure exists independently of his substantive philosophical commitments. Before concluding, I argue that the failure of Fromm's approach to social pathology to attain greater traction might be due to contingent aspects of his biography, rather than limitations in his scholarship.

In light of Fromm's approach, I reaffirm my central argument: the need to rectify the restrictive, recognition-derived framing of social pathology which dominates contemporary

---

[101] In a larger project it would be productive to bring Fromm's framing of alienation into dialogue with Jaeggi's (2016) more recent formulation. Fromm is more 'orthodox' in terms of his Marxian heritage, while Jaeggi's sits apart from Fromm's normative-essentialist-Marxist-humanist foundations.

[102] While I briefly engage with Fromm's broader philosophical commitments, due to limitations in space this can only be done incompletely. The core submission offered by this chapter is to point to the displaced utility of Fromm's social-theoretical infrastructure for furthering pathology diagnosing social criticism.

scholarship. This would enable Fromm's meritorious insights to be incorporated within a revitalised, 'undomesticated', social theoretical arsenal (Thompson M J, 2016). Only then will Critical Theorists be able to engage with the true breadth of the pathologies of the social.

The social pathology of normalcy: a sympathetic reconstruction

Fromm's framework is comprised of three distinct conceptual insights:

a) an understanding of the social world as pathological insofar as its conditions serve to alienate subjects from their true nature, and the wider social reality, conditions which are incommensurable with the requirements of 'normative humanism',

b) where individual subjects suffer from 'socially patterned defects' to the extent that they are incapable of realising their own alienation, and,

c) where such a pathological state is reinforced as 'the norm' through the process of 'consensual validation'; a social dynamic exists which drags potentially critical minds into conformity.

While these three insights each carry immense social theoretical value, Fromm's conception of social pathology achieves its real potency through their seamless aggregation. The three framings are presented with varying emphases across Fromm's *oeuvre*. While one can locate traces of the ideas of normative humanism, consensual validation, and socially patterned defects across *The Sane Society* (1955), *Beyond the Chains of Illusion* (1962), and Fromm's lecture series *The Pathology of Normalcy* (1991), there is no single grand exposé uniting the three analytics. Fromm's failure to unite the core insights constituting the pathology of normalcy in an accessible singular work must be a substantial factor in the comparable lack of attention paid to his conception of social pathology.

Objectively sub-optimal social conditions

Originating in a lesser known paper, 'Individual and Social Origins of Neurosis' (1944), but most extensively articulated in *The Sane Society*, Fromm is famous for his strident submission of a 'normative humanism' (Fromm, 1963: 12).[103] For Fromm, there are 'right and wrong' solutions to the question of 'human existence' (Fromm, 1963: 14).[104] Advancing the need for a 'science of

---

[103] For an extended sympathetic discussion on normative humanism see Michael J Thompson's (2017) 'Normative Humanism as Redemptive Critique'.

[104] Fromm's universality, his normative-essentialism, and his clear rejection of social constructivist accounts all place him in opposition to post-modern and post-structuralist approaches to the social theory (Ratner, 2014). I engage with these concerns later in the chapter.

man', Fromm submitted that there exists discoverable 'laws which govern ... mental and emotional functioning' (Fromm, 1963: 12). Through extended interdisciplinary investigation, such optimal conditions could be discovered. For Fromm, there were certain societies that were fundamentally more or less compatible with these requirements of a happy and meaningful ('sane') human life (Fromm, 1963, 1979, 1983, 2010). Such an analysis was presented as simultaneously normative, 'objective' and universal. Fromm's corpus built towards his 'road to sanity' (Jeffries, 2017: 293), demonstrating the 'objective' inferiority of our current form of social existence, and presenting the possibility of a new, 'saner' form of post-capitalist community. The core of Fromm's framing of pathological normalcy is his analysis that the accepted, 'normal' objective social conditions are found-wanting, relative to the attainable superior conditions dictated by normative humanism (Funk, 2010: 9).[105] To reiterate, Fromm's foundational insight is that the current, 'material', social world, in its everyday, 'normal' functioning, is incompatible with the conditions of normative humanism: it prohibits social subjects from living a meaningful and happy life. This can be read as the primary condition of Fromm's diagnosis of pathological normalcy: that there are objective social realities present in societies' routine, 'normal' operations which can objectively be deemed pathological or insane and which induce neuroses and alienation. In *The Sane Society* Fromm also describes the subject as suffering from 'insanity' as a result of the pathological state of the social order.[106]

One cannot overstress the import of Groddeck's (1929, 1977, 2012, 2013) work to Fromm's approach; one could argue that it was Groddeck's (1929, 1977) particular fusion of sociology and Freudian psychoanalysis that inspired Fromm's theoretical infrastructure and his substantive social theory (Biancoli, 1995). Fromm is directly following Groddeck's (1913, 1929, 1977) reading of Freud when he argues that objective social conditions precipitate 'social neurosis', and, therefore, it is the objective social conditions which require critique (Fromm, 1983: 56; Biancoli, 1995).[107] For Groddeck, clearly drawing on Freud,

> ... many illnesses are the product of people's lifestyles. If one wants to heal them, one has to change a patient's way of life; only in very few cases can the illness itself be tackled through so called specifica [sic] (Will, 1984: 22).

---

[105] The substantive content of these conditions was to be explored through Fromm's 'Science of Man', an attempt to combine the insights of sociology and biology in a 'total' analysis (Fromm, 1963: 14). Such a project never achieved sufficient institutional traction.

[106] While this analysis is particularly prominent in *The Sane Society*, in other texts and lectures Fromm does not refer to social subjects as 'insane', rather the subject is described as being 'alienated' or suffering from 'neuroses'. When commenting on Fromm's complete works it is better to speak of the 'insanity' of the social order rather than the 'insanity' of the social subject.

[107] Freud argued in *Civilisation and its Discontents* that the fundamental 'system of civilization' has become 'neurotic' (Freud, 1953: 142).

It is through Groddeck's (1977) reading of Freud as necessitating a critical sociology that Fromm develops his psycho-analytic-sociological paradigm. It is the 'insane society' that produces insane subjects; society itself that is pathological: 'mens sana in societate sana' (Fromm, 2010: 86).[108]

The cornerstone of Fromm's framing of 'pathological normalcy' is that the objective social order is found wanting: it fails to provide the conditions necessary for 'sane' human life as determined by normative humanism. Drawing on Freud, Fromm argues that it is our social conditions which precipitate dominant neuroses and insanities (and other non-medicalised impediments to our general wellbeing).[109] Uniting Freud and Marx, psychoanalysis and critical sociology, Fromm argues that a particular component of the objective social reality, *the capitalist economic system*, is overwhelmingly responsible for precipitating a particular form of 'insanity' and discomfort: alienation. The pervasiveness of late capitalism means that such alienation is not restricted to one's employment. Rather, with the subsumptive commodifying and 'abstractifying' rationalities of the market, man is constantly alienated from himself, from his fellows, and from his capacity to live itself.[110]

A socially patterned defect: where individuals are unaware of their own alienation

While the foundational diagnosis of Fromm's 'pathological normalcy' is that the objective conditions of capitalist society are contradictory to the demands of normative humanism, Fromm's account contains two further meritorious insights. For Fromm this 'pathological' condition developed into a normalcy because social processes acculturate subjects to consider their daily pathological reality both 'unproblematic' and 'normal'. Expressed most simply, an essential part of Fromm's framing of 'pathological normalcy' is that, at the level of the individual subject, due to a 'socially patterned defect' (Fromm, 1963: 15), *subjects are unaware of their own alienation*. There is no personal, individual realisation, let alone recognition, that the social order is 'insane', that is, antithetical to the optimal conditions for human sociality and well-being.

---

[108] I translate this from Latin as 'a healthy mind requires a healthy society'.
[109] See Honneth's (2014: 698) commentary on Mitscherlich and Freud for a further discussion on this point.
[110] In a broader project it would be interesting to connect this with Bertell Ollman's *Alienation* (1971). As with Jaeggi's (2016) more recent account, Ollman is less orthodox in his Marxism than Fromm, however he is more invested in a dialectical approach to understanding alienation (Ollman, 2003). For Ollman it is perhaps clearer to say that the pathological alienation of capitalist society arises from the inability of capitalist society to satisfactorily subflate the contradiction that capitalist alienation is more clearly understood as the problematic lack of unalienation (Ollman, 2003).

To further this analysis, Fromm again unites Freud and Marx. Social subjects are held to be complicit in their own alienation insofar as they perpetuate illusions about their own conditions; hence the title of Fromm's *Beyond The Chains of Illusion*. As Fromm states towards the start of the work, for both Marx and Freud,

> man lives with illusions because these illusions make the misery of real life bearable (Fromm, 1983: 15).

'Man' (or better, 'people') are complicit in deluding themselves so they may forget their 'dependency, ... [their] alienation, [their] ... slavery to the economy' (Fromm, 1983: 14). Finding similar cause again in Marx and Freud, Fromm thus presents 'truth' as a weapon to induce social change.[111] The animus of his work thus becomes to 'enable [the reader] ... to wake up and act as a free man' (Fromm, 1983: 16). Fromm makes a broader, anthropological point, which, while factually dubious, underscores his conviction:

> all the human race has achieved, spiritually and materially, it owes to the destroyers of illusion and to the seekers of reality (Fromm, 1983: 152).

Quoting Marx's chiasmus liberally, Fromm elaborates, man's

> demand to give up the illusions about ... [his] condition is the demand to give up a condition which needs illusions (Marx, 1959: 16; c.f. Fromm, 1983: 105).

Thus, 'truth', and an awareness of the latent desire for truth, can be wielded as a weapon of praxis to achieve social change.[112] Uniting insights from Marx and Freud, but drawing more extensively on Marx,[113] Fromm's analysis is that pathological normalcy is re-inscribed through illusions functioning as 'opiate(s) against the socially patterned defect' (Fromm, 1963: 17). In the words of Fromm's former student, and biographer, Rainer Funk,

> the fact that we do not experience the emptying and devaluation of the subject, as well as the dependency on the market as something abnormal anymore is a central indication for what Fromm ultimately calls 'the pathology of normalcy' (Funk, 2000: 11).

---

[111] This is reminiscent of the more problematic Lenin quote, 'The Marxist doctrine is omnipotent because it is true' (1977: 21). To restate, this thesis prefers to champion pathology diagnosis as a methodology, and to connect this with the Critical Theoretical approach of exploring possibilities for immanent-transcendence. I am less invested in the claims to the explicit 'truth' of any social pathology diagnosis, this seems potentially politically suspect. Reading Fromm charitably, we can see traces of the methodological aspect of the search for truth in his methodology, the desire to sweep away illusions. This is not to state what will be discovered will be an unmediated truth.

[112] For Honneth (2007c), drawing on Freud, there is a foundational, even anthropological desire to grasp for the truth of our conditions, as a means of overcoming neuroses. Honneth appeals to such libidinal cathexis to provides animus for Critical Theory itself (Honneth, 2007b, 2007c).

[113] Fromm repeatedly suggests Marx is the superior thinker of the two, he states at one point: Freud 'did not reach the heights of Marx' (Fromm, 1983: 12).

A dynamic of consensual validation: where mass acceptance of the norm serves to inhibit critique

The third constituent of Fromm's framework is a dynamic of 'consensual validation' (Fromm, 1963: 14). This is expressed most extensively in the second chapter of *The Sane Society* (1963: 12-21), yet there are references to this dynamic in Fromm's lecture series, *The Pathology of Normalcy* (2010). The essential argument here is that, within the social order, dynamics arise which retard critical awareness of the pathological norm. As Fromm argues,

> What is so deceptive about the state of mind of the members of a society is the "consensual validation" of their concepts. It is naively assumed that the fact that the majority of people share certain ideas or feelings proves the validity of these ideas and feelings. Nothing is further from the truth (Fromm, 1963: 14).

Further,

> Just as there is "folie a deux" there is "folie a millions". The fact that millions of people share the same vices does not make these vices virtues. The fact that they share so many errors does not make the errors to be truths, and the fact that millions of people share the same forms of mental pathology does not make these people sane (Fromm, 1963: 15).

Yet, the fact that millions of people do share the same errors, do suffer from the same vices, *does* serve to impede critical awareness of the broader pathological conditions. In one of his earliest lectures at *The New School*, Fromm related Wells' (1904) tale, *The Country of the Blind*, to prove this point (Fromm, 2010: 17).[114] Paraphrasing Fromm's own paraphrasing of Wells, the story proceeds thus: a healthy stranger lost in a rainforest stumbles into a village home to an isolated tribe. Due to a genetic defect among the population, the local population is blind. They have clearly defined smooth, silky skin growing over their eyelids, and none of the tribe has ever heard of sight. In the country of the blind, the one-eyed man is not king, rather he is an insane lunatic, with his phantasmal, psychotic visions. Further, he is stigmatised for the unseemly nature of his pupils, rather than the desirable, smooth skin to which the populace are accustomed. The ease with which the 'hysteria of hate' (Fromm, 1983: 6) was whipped up against the hapless migrant is furthered by the dynamic of consensual validation. All of those present in the village, save the one, weary traveller, are mutually reassured of their factual accuracy, and remain ignorant to the possibility they are living a less than optimal human existence. Even if the stranger was exceptionally persuasive, and unprecedently biologically insightful, people are unable to simply 'look at the facts' (Fromm, 1963: 3). The social subjects' understanding remains *deeply socially located;* for Fromm, 'individual psychology is [thus] fundamentally social psychology' (Fromm, 1941: 20).

---

[114] Fromm also presents a secondary anecdote (Fromm, 2010: 18). Paraphrasing, Fromm tells of a man who goes to the doctor and, contextualising his systems, details his morning routine. He incidentally details how he brushes his teeth and vomits every morning. For the patient, accustomed as he is to daily retching, this is the normalcy, and neither merits concern, nor non-incidental comment. He is only aware of the pathological nature of his newer, in his mind, more troubling symptoms.

While 'consensual validation as such has no bearing on reason or mental health' (Fromm, 1963: 14-15), it is accompanied by dynamics which serve to protect the subject from developing a personal manifestation of the social neurosis.[115] Using the example of Calvinism, Fromm suggests societies develop in such a manner that the individual's commitment to the polity's pathological demands is ultimately elevated, rather than obscured. Not only is the social subject, while suffering from a 'socially patterned defect', 'not aware' of this reality; but 'his very defect … [is thus] … raised … [as] … a virtue' (Fromm, 1963: 15). For A Thompson, this is best characterised as 'a process of dynamic adaption between social structures and individual psyche' (Thompson A, 2009: 101). In Fromm's words,

> What he may have lost in richness and in a genuine feeling of happiness, is made up by the security of fitting in with the rest of mankind – *as he knows them* (Fromm, 1963: 15).

Thus, a crucial aspect of the pathology of normalcy is the extent to which capitalist dynamics *are the normalcy*: the social subject draws succour from compliance with the normal. Pathological normalcy is harder to overthrow because its status as normalcy comforts and supports the subjects to accommodate the polity's pathological defects.

For Fromm, then, 'the irrationality of human mass behaviour', evinced though the proclivity of the social subject to conform to any norm (Fromm, 1983: 8), is an antecedent, almost an anthropological, flaw. Fromm's manumission of the social subject from the chains of illusion thus necessitates inducing a primary scepticism to 'common thought' (Fromm, 1983: 14): the social subject must no longer concede to the irrationality of consensual validation.

Two years after *Beyond the Chains of Illusion* was published, Stanley Kubrick's black-comedy *Dr. Strangelove* was premiered. With its immortal line from President Muffley (Peter Sellers), 'Gentlemen, you can't fight in here! This is the war room!' (Kubrick, 1964), one can sense the extent to which Fromm's work may have had a particular resonance in Cold War America. What aesthetic critics may deem the 'dramatic irony' of Muffley's line, Fromm may have seen as an epitomic symptom of pathological normalcy. For Fromm, the solution to the siren call of consensual validation, paraphrasing Marx once again, is: *De Omnibus Dubitandum Est* [above all, one must doubt] (McLellan, 1985: 457).[116]

---

[115] Fromm implicitly presents this as essential to the analytic, but one can clearly foresee scenarios where such a dynamic could exist, without such additional palliatives.

[116] Marx was given a set of questions to answer by his daughters Jenny and Laura. In addition to revealing his favourite food was fish, he revealed that his favourite motto was 'De omnibus dubitandum' (Marx [1865]). This quote, of course, is a paraphrasing of Descartes.

The centrality, and social-theoretical utility, of Fromm's framing of alienation

Jeffries argues that Marx's concept of alienation is central to Fromm's diagnosis: 'the overcoming of alienation' (Fromm, 2010: 85) is the true momentum propelling the reader along Fromm's 'road to sanity' (Jeffries, 2017: 293). Drawing on Marx, Fromm's insight is that,

> what is good for the function of today's economic system proceeds to be damaging to the maintenance of man's mental health (Funk, 2010: 9-10).

For Funk, Fromm is explicit in his analysis,

> current production methods and ... [the] psychic efforts to conform ... [with the] ... demands of the current economy ... make ... [man] psychically ill (Funk, 2010: 9).[117]

It is worth tracing the development of Fromm's thought here. Fromm's focus on alienation, precipitated by the economic system of 'abstractification'[118] (Fromm, 2010: 63) is most extensively espoused in *Marx's Concept of Man* and *Beyond the Chains of Illusion*. In these works, Fromm locates his understanding within the left-Hegelian imaginary. It is well known that for Hegel, God exists in man, and that history is the process of God returning to himself. For the 'Young Hegelian' Feuerbach, *pace* Hegel, 'God' represents man's own powers. For Feuerbach (2008 [1841]), as espoused in *The Essence of Christianity,* the more humanity ascribes its power to God, the weaker man becomes. For Marx, the same occurs with alienation in the material realm through the processes of capitalist production:

> ... the worker becomes poorer the more wealth he produces and the more his production increases in power and extent (Marx, 1961: 95; c.f. Fromm, 1983: 42).

This...

> follow[s] from the fact that the worker is related to the *product of his labor* as to an *alien* object. For it is clear on this presupposition that the more the worker expends himself in work, the more powerful becomes the world of objects which he creates in face of himself, the poorer he becomes in his inner life and the less he belongs to himself: it is just the same as in religion (Marx, 1961: 95-96; c.f. Fromm, 1983: 42-43).

Further:

> The worker puts his life into the object and his life then belongs no longer to himself but to the object. The greater his activity, therefore, the less he possesses ... The *alienation* of the worker in his product means not only that his labour becomes an object, assumes an external existence, but that it exists independently, outside himself, that it stands opposed to him as an autonomous power. The life which he has given to the object sets itself against him as an alien and hostile force (Marx, 1961: 95-96; and c.f. Fromm, 1983: 43).

For Marx, and for Fromm, the worker is alienated not just 'from the products' but also from 'the *process'* of production (Fromm, 1983: 43). Alienation thus appears 'within *productive activity'*

---

[117] Such an approach seems to closely foreshadow Honneth's (2004) conception of 'organized self-realization'. It is further telling of Fromm's contemporary intellectual ostracision that Honneth does not acknowledge, or engage with Fromm in his framing, despite their striking similarities (Honneth, 2004).

[118] Interesting to note the clear similarity to Lukacs' (1972) work on 'reification', yet Fromm's decision to use the term 'abstractification' instead. I have failed to find any further scholarship on this point.

(Marx, 1961: 99; c.f. Fromm, 1983: 43) and excludes man from productive activity. Fromm extends this analysis, arguing Marx is concerned with 'man's alienation from life, from himself, and from his fellow man' (Fromm, 1983: 44). Citing liberally from the *Economic and Philosophical Manuscripts*, Fromm utilises Marx to argue that the capitalist system of production produces a totally alienated subjectivity: alienated from himself, from the process of production, from his fellow humans, so that 'life itself appears only as a *means of life*' (c.f. Fromm, 1983: 44; Marx, 1961: 101). Fromm reads Marx as 'proceed[ing] to the concept of man's alienation from himself, his fellowmen, and from nature': 'from the concept of alienated work' (Fromm, 1983: 43). The pathological material, political-economic logics and realities of capitalism precipitate pathological cognitive states.

To state it explicitly: such alienation is held to be in breach of the conditions of normative-humanism and is therefore a social pathology. Again, in direct contrast to the recognition approaches' neo-idealism, Fromm's diagnosis of alienation is explicitly linked to the economic system of production. The psychic phenomena of alienation is a direct result of the objective social conditions. To support this position, Fromm again turns to Marx, this time to *The German Ideology*:

> As long as a cleavage exists between the particular and the common interest man's own deed becomes an alien power opposed to him, which enslaves him (Marx and Engels, 1939: 220; Fromm, 1983: 44).

Fromm explicitly locates the cause of such alienation in the 'contemporary mode of production' (Fromm, 1983: 56). Alienation[119] can only be overcome through 'the complete change of the economic-social constellation' (Fromm, 1983: 56). For Fromm, the market 'has reached such proportions' that 'all participants have been moulded by it' that 'all experiences' have 'become abstract as commodities' (Fromm, 2010: 63).[120] Jeffries paraphrases Fromm thus: the 'external social structures' of the market are pathologically 'shaping the inner self' (Jeffries, 2017: 292). It is this crucial awareness that is fundamentally lacking in the neo-idealist, recognition-cognitive diagnoses of social pathology.

In Fromm's analysis, the foundational social pathology, the driving force perpetuating conditions anathema to normative humanism, is the capitalist mode of production. Thus, *la Maladie du Siecle*, the cognitive 'estrangement of man from his own humanity' (Fromm, 1983: 56), can only be rectified through a foundational change in the rationality of the economic

---

[119] See my later comments on Fromm's broader eschatology. Here, alienation is used in an immanent, material context.
[120] In such analysis one can see the prefiguration of Habermas' (1984) understanding of the colonisation of the 'lifeworld' by the logics of the 'system' in his *Theory of Communicative Action*.

system. For Ratner, it is clear that for Fromm's diagnosed pathological normalcy to be 'cured' there needs to be foundational changes to 'macro-cultural forces' (Ratner, 2014: 300).

As established, today's dominant framing of social pathology presents a troublingly ossifying dichotomy between social maladies existing 'in the world', and those existing 'in the head' of the social subject (Freyenhagen, 2015: 136). To repeat, today's mainstream scholarship views merely the latter, recognition-cognitive maladies, as social pathologies (Zurn, 2011). Further, as M J Thompson's critique of neo-Idealism elaborates, today's approach fails to engage sufficiently with the impact of social structural logics on the capacities of the social subject. These artificial restrictions dogging today's scholarship are transcended through Fromm's three central analytics:

a) alienation as a condition induced by objective social conditions ('world'), which is

b) unintelligible to the pathological, 'insane', social subject who suffers from a socially patterned defect ('cognitive');

c) said defect is further re-inscribed by the siren allure of the modalities of consensual validation ('world' and 'cognitive').

Fromm's substantive diagnosis is thus simply one of alienation: he writes 'we are aliens to ourselves' (Fromm, 2010: 46), alienation is *the* sickness of man' (Fromm, 1983: 45), and that 'every neurosis can be considered an outcome of alienation' (Fromm, 1983: 53). Fromm thus develops and deploys his secondary analytics, consensual validation and socially patterned defects, to further his diagnosis of alienation. Cognitive and material are united, seamlessly reproducing each other. As with Jaeggi's (2016) phenomenologically grounded study of alienation, Fromm's diagnosis portrays how a critique of social-structural logics discloses the helplessness and despondency of the capitalist subject. The pathological material logics precipitate a pathologically impaired mental state. This process is seamlessly captured through Fromm's framing of alienation.

Such comments are warranted to demonstrate the centrality of alienation, and its *Aufheben,* to Fromm's broader work, not merely its dominance in his united psycho-analytic and critical sociological scholarship. This is not intended as an advocation of the sentiments of Fromm's eschatology, or his metaphysics: the submission here is merely that Fromm provides a stimulating substantive philosophy, consideration of which can help revitalise social pathology scholarship. While this chapter thus presents the merit of engaging with Fromm's substantive considerations, the primary attachment here, as established, is to his social theoretical infrastructure.

Thus far, the chapter has presented a highly sympathetic engagement with Fromm's work. Yet, today, Fromm's scholarship is often excluded from discussions of social pathology on various, *prima facie,* highly damaging counts. The next section acknowledges the manifold critiques of Fromm's philosophy, and indeed, the multiple critiques levelled at his social theory and his psychoanalytic insights.[121]

The Problems faced when engaging with Fromm's work today[122]

Fromm's work may seem 'almost archaic' at first encounter, both stylistically and substantively (Thompson A, 2009: 25). This section presents three areas where Fromm scholarship sits at variance from contemporary theoretical insights. Having outlined these areas of divergence I expiate Fromm's core social-theoretical infrastructure. In crude summary, progressive academics may be 'wary' engaging with Fromm (Thompson A, 2009: 20) because:

   a) Fromm routinely uses gendered language, think of *Marx's Concept of Man* or, *Man for Himself*. There is a recurring concern that this is indicative of broader, problematic patriarchal complicities.

   b) Perhaps even more problematically, Fromm's substantive theories are held to be at odds with the dominant presumptions of ethical-cultural relativism intrinsic to the post-modern, post-structural academy (Ratner, 2014). Thus, to the contemporary eye, Fromm's work may seem both dated, and flawed. His unrepentant universalism and ethical partisanship (*a la* normative humanism) falls into sharp relief against the background of the extended crisis of normativity (Butler, Laclau, and Zizek, 2000; Honneth, 1999, 2005).

Drawing on Thompson (2009), the submission here is that one can extricate Fromm's insightful analysis from his problematic, only *incidentally* patriarchal, lexicon. In response to the post-modern and post-structural critiques of Fromm's (apparent) universality, two responses are presented. First, Fromm's philosophy could be redeemable despite his ethical partisanship and his unchecked claims to universality, through a turn to Honneth's 'patch' of a weak formal anthropology. Second, even if Fromm's philosophical commitments are untenable in light of the insights of post-modern and post-structuralist scholarship, Fromm's social theoretical infrastructure can be extricated from his more divisive theses.

---

[121] And indeed, with the psychoanalytic orthodoxy more broadly. See my engagement with Selby (1993), Butler (1997), Miller (1974), Lacan (1975) and Zupančič (2017).

[122] Obviously, this list is not exhaustive. One might also comment on how Fromm's scholarship has been displaced by left-scholarship too, for instance by the rise of Althusserian anti-humanist Marxism.

Gender critiques of Fromm

Fromm repeatedly speaks of 'man' where his meaning is more broadly 'people' or 'humanity'. It is disconcerting for the contemporary reader, and a source of conflicting critical discussion (Burston, 1991; Thompson A, 2009: 25-26). While such a charge could be levelled at most thinkers of the socio-philosophical canon (Alanen and Witt, 2004), the critical literature surrounding Fromm focuses on this theme with particular interest, hence my engagement here. Further, the purpose of my analysis in this section is to demonstrate the extent to which Fromm's scholarship is needlessly negated, hence my engagement with what may seem to some, *prima facie*, superficial critiques. My submission is that, ultimately, such charges are indeed overstated.

Thompson explicitly addresses the issue of Fromm's '"sexist" language', commenting that it seems 'at odds with his humanist principles' (Thompson A, 2009: 25). While she does not argue for negating this possibility entirely, she does raise three points worthy of consideration.

First, Fromm came to English from a German background. In German the word 'Mensch', while often grammatically gendered male, has a meaning closer to 'humanity': it undoubtedly sounds less jarring to the contemporary ear. Similarly, the German 'Mann' functions in German closer to the English word 'one' rather than 'man'. Thompson comments that there is simply no perfect translation, no 'appropriate English term' (Thompson A, 2009: 25). For Fromm, his use of 'Man' is as close as he can get to his intended German 'Mensch'. One can argue that his analytic infrastructure was developed independently from this incidentally patriarchal prose; a result of the relative limitations of the English language.

Second, A. Thompson (2009) points to Fromm's (1976) own discussion on this point in his *To Have or To Be?* Fromm claims that he explicitly sought to 'restore [Mensch's] non-sexual meaning' (Fromm, 1979: 10). For Thompson, it is worth reading Fromm's own words on this topic. Engaging with this argument with Neil Wilson's (1959) 'spirit of charitable interpretation', one should perhaps read Fromm as consciously aware of this lacuna in English prose, and as seeking to surmount it, rather than reinforce it. Admittedly, not all scholars advance the same degree of charity (Thompson A, 2009).

Third, Thompson raises the point that 'this usage was common in [Fromm's] time' (Thompson A, 2009: 25). When the problematic prose is incidental to Fromm's argumentation (if one accepts the reasonable position that it is as close to the German 'Mensch' as Fromm could reach) it would be uncharitable to judge the work anachronistically. Just as Darwin's (1871) *The Descent of Man* utilises gendered language, the substantial content of his manuscript is irrefutably worthy of engagement; the same follows for Fromm.

While I consider that these three positions respond adequately to the charge of Fromm's use of gendered language, feminist engagements with Fromm, and with psychoanalysis more broadly, have suggested a deeper complicity in patriarchal structures (Miller, 1974). Recall Lacan's pronouncement that 'there is no such thing as woman' (Lacan, 1975: 68). While this extends beyond the scope of the current chapter, in brief response I point the reader towards Selby's (1993) article, *Psychoanalysis as a Critical Theory of Gender*. I do this to reinforce that a substantial debate exists on this point, and that many in the academy successfully reconcile the patriarchal complicity of psychoanalytic orthodoxy with its undeniable insights for critical social theory (Butler, 1997).

'The Road to Sanity' and Normative Humanism: Ethical partisanship and Universality[123]

Forms of social pathology diagnosis which are predicated on partisan ethics are now justifiably subject to intense philosophical suspicion (Honneth, 1999, 2015). Such ethically derived critique is controversial in today's conditions of normative crisis (Thompson M J, 2014). There remains no philosophical consensus upon acceptable foundations from which to ground ideas of the good life (Honneth, 1999, 2005). Fromm's commitment to the contrary presents a significant challenge for contemporary engagements with his work (Thompson M J, 2014).

Remember that core to Fromm's diagnosis of pathological normalcy is his contention that the existent conditions of society fall foul of the objectively essential social conditions needed for a 'sane' and meaningful life. For Fromm such conditions were ascertainable through normative humanism, and substantively articulable through 'the science of man'. Such a methodology is an explicit invocation of a partisan ethics: Fromm's account here is predicated on his assertion that he has access to a superior ethics.

Fromm commits a second cardinal sin in the eyes of social-constructivists: unjustifiable universalism. Not only does Fromm suggest that society X is failing, but he also presents it as failing *for all human beings*. Further, he suggests there are essential human characteristics which are identical across time and place (the underlying core of his normative humanism). Such a

---

[123] While the dominant critiques of Fromm's work occur from a broadly social-constructivist post-modern framework (Ratner, 2014) and it is thus to those that I respond, one could sidestep such critiques with a strident defence of a critical realist framework. Indeed Vandenberghe (2013) has written extensively about the untapped potential of using a critical realist account to further critical social theory.

position is fundamentally incompatible with both strong social-constructivism[124] and the basic precepts of post-modernist thought. Writing before post-structuralist and post-modernist insights, Fromm felt comfortable presenting his universalist and ethically partisan theories without such considered justifications.[125]

For Ratner, Fromm's work is thus needlessly discarded today in its entirety, for his *oeuvre* sits in opposition to the prevailing 'constructivist-relativism' (Ratner, 2014: 301). Today's 'diversity-constructivist' normalcy makes it impossible to pass judgement on the conditions needed for the good life (Ratner, 2014: 301). Ratner gives the example that it is now philosophically unjustifiable to consider a morbidly obese individual to be suffering from a form of pathology (Ratner, 2014: 301), as someone living an objectively impeded existence (O'Hara and Gregg, 2012). For the committed post-structuralist, attuned to a world lacking normative anchoring, one cannot comment that such an individual is suffering from a pathology, that they are objectively suffering from a condition impeding their quality of life. Today, such an approach to 'objective biological illness' would be held to be both politically dangerous and philosophically unjustifiable (Honneth, 2014a: 684). For Foucault, such 'pathologising' discourse is utilised predominantly to bring forth subjectivities for 'disciplining' (Dreyfus and Rabinow, 1982: 173) and to perpetuate and legitimate governmentality. For Foucault, Fromm's framing of normative humanism would be pernicious and philosophically unsound: a mere reflection of the dominant discursively constructed value-horizon of Fromm's contingent historical moment, rather than a guide to objective reality. Even more troublingly for Foucault, such insight, while academically worthless,[126] could ultimately prove of utility for pernicious authoritative assemblies, who could mobilise such sentiments to further coercive governmentality.

While the post-modern[127] insight served to displace the philosophical acceptability of ethical partisanship and universality, it failed to institute an alternate conception of subjectivity, attuned to its foundational insights. Rather, the academic mainstream today holds to a

---

[124] There is an increasingly articulate counter-position emerging amongst psychologists. Pinker's (2003) *The Blank Slate* provides a strong critique of the dominant social constructivism, and argues for the existence of an accessible, and universal, human nature.

[125] Fromm comes closest to such a justification in his *Marx's Concept of Man,* however, to subject such an account to the insights of post-structuralism would be both anachronistic and unproductive. Fromm's submissions here are best understood as located within the concerns of his time.

[126] Of course, it is not merely Foucault and post-structuralists who would reject Fromm's normative humanism, and the methodology of the 'science of man'. M J Thompson (2014) comments how Weberian sociologists, for example, would be critical of Fromm here, in that he risks the non-separation of 'fact' and 'value'. That said, it would seem arbitrary to direct any impassioned challenge at Fromm on this account, considering said is/ought separation is programmatically breached by the entire 'First Generation of Critical Theory'.

[127] Admittedly, I am using these terms rather loosely. A larger project would have more space to disaggregate post-structuralist and post-modernist critiques, however, I suggest that for the purposes of this chapter, the desired argument (that Fromm's theoretical infrastructure can be expiated) can made without such an extended discussion.

'subjectivity [that] is autonomous, personal, and self-directed' (Ratner, 2014: 301); a view entirely opposed by post-structural, and Critical Theory. Ironically, today, the dominant 'position that denies the very existence of pathology is rooted in a broad social philosophy of individual freedom, authenticity, personhood, ageing, and subjectivity' (Ratner, 2014: 301). I concur with Ratner that such a 'social philosophy is essentially post-modernist and neoliberal' (Ratner, 2014: 301). In light of such developments, I turn to Honneth's conception of a 'weak-formal anthropology' (Honneth, 2007a: 42) as a means to square the circle of the unjustifiability of, but the essential need to, base our critique in a normativity to be able to conduct social pathology diagnosing critique.[128]

Honneth believes that social theorists can operate within the horizons of 'a weak formal anthropology' to facilitate philosophically justifiable engagement on 'conceptions of ethical life' providing that such an anthropology is sufficiently abstract (Honneth, 2007a). If the weak formal anthropology remains suitably open, the post-structuralist charge of privileging particular visions of the good life can be temporarily displaced (Honneth, 2007a). The normative challenges are neither solved nor obviated, rather they are 'patched' to enable the crucial continuance of critique. For Foucault scholars Dreyfus and Rabinow (1982), the post-structuralist normative critique holds most strongly against 'meta-theory'.[129] The challenge then is to maintain a weak formal anthropology that is substantive enough to enable social pathology diagnosis, yet weak enough to avoid the charge of bloated meta-theoretical universalism. Such an approach may work as effectively when applied to Fromm's account as it does when utilised by Honneth. Thus, to substantially expiate the charge that Fromm's work unjustifiably makes universalising and ethically partisan commitments, one may retro-actively redact Fromm's formal conception of normative humanism, and instead displace it with a weak-formal anthropological account of normative humanism. For Honneth, at least, and for those who follow in his intellectual footsteps, such a charge of normative and universalising untenability would then be temporarily abated.[130]

---

[128] The reader may have thought it more amenable to turn to Habermas' (1998) discursive justification of the content of (moral) norms; however, following M J Thompson (2014), I consider such an approach unsatisfactory. While Habermas' presentation purports to determine the objective content of morality, it fails to extend beyond the confines of the merely cognitive. Habermas' solution seems insufficient for my purposes here, for it fails to determine any ontologically grounded objectivity to claim making *beyond the structure of language*. Further, such an approach could rightfully be critiqued as neo-Idealistic, insofar as the linguistic dimension is held to contain emancipatory potential untarnished by the structural modalities of the system; modalities Habermas himself earlier argued were colonising the communicative sphere.

[129] See the interview with Foucault at the end off *Beyond Structuralism and Hermeneutics*. To some extent this is a development of Foucault's (1975) *Discipline and Punish*, but I find this figuration of particular clarity.

[130] Such an approach would sit comfortably with the work of Durkin (2014) and Wilde (2004) who suggest that Fromm's account is already sufficiently 'thin' to counter the social-constructionist critique.

This approach would, however, fail to satisfy committed social-constructivists. To such a critique, I offer a secondary reply. The purpose of my engagement with Fromm is to articulate the strength of his social theoretical infrastructure. This social-theoretical infrastructure can be used to great impact for critical social theory, shorn of Fromm's *philosophical content*. Indeed, one may isolate Fromm's foundational methods, his incidental language, and his eschatology, from the social theoretical infrastructure at the core of his conception of social pathology.

Fromm's normative humanism can be displaced by an alternate basis for ethical critique. For instance, one could submit that the present social order evinces immanent contradictions (which is already the basic methodological commitment for most Critical Theory). From such a foundation, the two other essential features of Fromm's framing are: a) that the social body has a dynamic in existence of consensual validation so that the social body is unaware of these internal contradictions; and b) that at an individual level subjects are unaware that they are living anything other than the fullest, most flourishing life, can effortlessly be integrated. Such an approach would retain the fundamental utility of Fromm's social theoretical infrastructure, while providing distance from the more troublesome aspects of Fromm's substantive philosophical convictions.

Ultimately, this chapter advocates the first of these two routes: Fromm's substantive submission can be of real potency and clarity. However, if the reader is not convinced by this earlier discussion, the foundational infrastructure Fromm provides can be seamlessly extricated. In either case, there are undeniable meritorious insights in Fromm's framing of social pathology that go unappreciated in the dominant contemporary literature.

Erich Fromm: 'The Forgotten Intellectual'

Before concluding, I wish to briefly argue that the failure of Fromm's approach to attain greater intellectual traction, and indeed his ultimate 'anathematization from Critical Theory' (Jeffries, 2017: 294) can be accounted for by the contingent facts of his biography. Fromm always felt at once removed from the society he described, while simultaneously invested in actively supporting its progressive development. This was as true of his relationship to 'Critical Theory' as it was to modernity writ large. As Thompson states,

> the theme of the *stranger*, of not quite belonging [,] and of alienation played an important part throughout his [own] life (Thompson A, 2009: 4).

After developing a reputation as an incisive interdisciplinary progressive thinker, Fromm was invited to join the Institute of Social Research. The origins of Fromm's eventual intellectual ostracision can be traced to his initial meeting with Theodor Adorno; from their very 'first acquaintance, Fromm … developed a marked aversion' to the philosopher (Funk, 2000: 97). Their mutual dislike is well charted (Thompson A, 2009: 12). Adorno effectively engineered Fromm's departure from the institute, which was but the first of multiple blows to Fromm's academic standing (Jeffries, 2017).

Perhaps the bloodiest of such contretemps was the 'bitter dispute' between Marcuse and Fromm that played out in the pages of *Dissent* in the second half of the 1950s (Jeffries, 2017: 289). For Witenberg, *The Dissent* debate damaged Fromm's reputation internationally, and with it, diminished substantive scholarly engagement with his work (Witenberg, 1997: 334). Marcuse's disagreement with Fromm was fundamentally over diverging readings of Freud (Jeffries, 2017: 289). In Jeffries' prose,

> Marcuse suggested that Fromm has smuggled capitalist values into his critique of the capitalist system (2017: 289).

For Burston, the brutality of the debate can be attributed to 'sibling rivalry' between Freud's heirs, both advancing revisions of Freud's foundational works (Burston, 1991: 226-227). The dispute was so intense that decades after, Fromm 'saw Marcuse on a train and studiously ignored him' (Jeffries, 2017: 294). The intense 'anathamezation [sic]' of Fromm by the core figures of the Frankfurt School can only have served to damage the standing of, and engagement with, his work as serious, considered scholarship (Jeffries, 2017: 294).

Beyond Critical Theoretical circles, Fromm's latter works were attacked by the psychoanalytic orthodoxy for a lack of focus on 'real life choices', considered an essential prerequisite for psychoanalytic application (Margolies, 1996). While Fromm's key works, especially *Fear Of Freedom* (1941)[131], *Man for Himself* (1947), *The Sane Society* (1955), *The Art of Loving* (1956), *Marx's Concept of Man* (1961), *Beyond the Chains of Illusion* (1962), *The Anatomy of Human Destructiveness* (1973) and *To Have or to Be?* (1976) were widely read, from the early 1960s he was increasingly seen as 'too provocative and disturbing to be readily assimilated into the analytic mainstream' (Burston and Olfman, 1996: 321). Despite the undeniable 'popularity of Fromm's work', the 'traditional academic and psychoanalytic' elite were 'wary' of Fromm's style and argumentation (Thompson A, 2009: 20).

Fromm died in 1980, aged 79, as 'the forgotten intellectual' (Braune, 2014: 3). Considering the extent of his output, and the devotion of his contemporary readership, that moniker remains apt today (Thompson M J, 2014). Indeed, a forthcoming paper in *The European Journal of Social Theory* presenting itself as articulating a complete typography of conceptions of social

---

[131] Published in the USA as *Escape from Freedom* in the same year. For consistency, in this thesis I stick to either untranslated or English titles.

pathology, fails to engage once with Fromm (Laitinen and Särkelä, 2019). For Witenberg, Fromm 'lost some influence by crossing academic boundaries' (Witenberg, 1997: 334), while for Jeffries the 'deck was stacked against him' from the very start (Jeffries, 2017: 294). Concurring with Jeffries, I argue that the merits of Fromm's scholarship have been underexplored through the impact of contingent life events, *in addition to* the current unfavourability of the sentiments he espoused following the post-modern and post-structural turns.

In keeping with his life, in death Fromm remains something of an outsider, neither fully integrated within the Critical Theoretical abode, nor fully excluded from it. Likewise, it is the case for his status relative to the psychoanalytic canon (Margolies, 1996). Through my presentation of this briefest of biographies, I hope to have established that Fromm scholarship may be lacking, not merely due to aversions to his substantive work, but additionally due to contingent, unfortunate facts of his life.

Conclusion

Fromm is at pains to stress his approach is 'not at all a psychological theory' (Fromm, 1983: 38).[132] With this insistence, one may read Fromm as prefiguring Freyenhagen's (2015) concerns over a dangerous 'cognitive/material' binary. *Social pathologies* are primarily *socially induced*, thus a meaningful analysis needs to extend far beyond the cognitive. Concurring with Fromm, the argument here is that a psychological/psychoanalytic theory absent a critical sociology risks becoming a futile endeavour. Such an approach hazards negating the centrality of social processes acting on the subject. A diagnosis of pathological normalcy must thus centre Fromm's essential, Groddeckian insight: 'individual psychology is [thus] fundamentally social psychology' (Fromm, 1941: 20). In *Beyond the Chains of Illusion*, Fromm (1983) implicitly acknowledges the lineage of this dictum to Marx's materialistic inversion of Hegel.

Fromm's framework offers real utility to the critical social theorist, and its exclusion from current conversations on, and typologies of, social pathology, is problematic. A Critical Theory seeking to transcend its current domesticated horizon could draw true support and vitality from Fromm's *oeuvre*. While Fromm's substantive social-theoretical and philosophical insights provide potent resources that can reinvigorate social pathology scholarship, it is Fromm's social theoretical infrastructure which this paper triumphs. The ossifying recognition-cognitive

---

[132] This particular phrasing seems to echo the introduction to Novak and Mandel's *The Marxist Theory of Alienation* (1973), where the co-authors comment immediately that alienation is neither primarily, nor solely, of psychic origin and location. Fromm's broader project can be read as a clear testimony to this fact; the pathology of normalcy has social structural origins.

approach to social pathology is effortlessly transcended in Fromm's analysis of alienation, which, as I draw out, is crucially connected to his social-structural critique. Through the seamless aggregation of an analysis of: a) sub-optimal social conditions, b) the manner in which such conditions are obscured at an individual level, and c) the social dynamics retarding critique, Fromm presents a framework which can be applied to patriarchal, neo-colonial as well as capitalist structures.

Fromm scholarship, while slowly growing, remains unduly limited. While the central tenets of his substantive philosophy may provide important resources for revitalising the diagnosis of social pathologies, the social theoretical infrastructure he provides is perhaps his most underappreciated legacy.

In Ratner's words,

Pathological normalcy leads to valuable ... insights for humanizing society on a practical, political level. Pathological normalcy provides us with a foundation for real social and psychological change (Ratner, 2014: 302).

Chapter Seven

Rethinking Recognition

Introduction

This chapter presents a way of incorporating the useful aspects of recognition theory as part of a broader social pathology diagnosing endeavour. As the preceding discussion has demonstrated (Chapters Four to Six), the dominant recognition perspective needlessly excludes potent theoretical approaches for engaging with social pathologies. The current recognition-derived framework fails to engage with the socio-cultural pathologies explored by Rousseau (Chapter Four), pathologies of reason (Chapter Five), or Fromm's work on pathological normalcy (Chapter Six). It is essential that any attempt to harbour the utility of the recognition approach as part of a broader 'polycentric and multilateral' Critical Theory does not replicate this needlessly exclusionary character (Fraser and Honneth, 2001: 209). In Fraser's words, the challenge is finding a way to incorporate the insights of recognition theory without 'putting all … [of our] eggs in one basket', i.e. without submitting to the exclusively recognition approach that Honneth advances (Fraser and Honneth, 2001: 205). The exercise at the heart of this chapter is to identify and extract the utility of the recognition theoretical framework, without being constrained, *pace* Honneth, to only viewing the pathologies of the social world through a recognition lens. This chapter thus presents a way of integrating a reformulated recognition framing within a raft of other approaches to pathology diagnosing social critique. While the *dominant* recognition approach is highly problematic, I consider it worth engaging with the broader tradition for two reasons: a) to capture the utility of recognition-derived approaches to social theory beyond the Honnethian approach, and b) to potentially bridge the divide between rival social-theoretical camps, bringing together scholars who embrace, and those who excoriate, the dominant recognition account (Harris, 2019).

This chapter has three sections. First, I briefly retrace the primary weaknesses inherent in mainstream recognition theoretical approaches and suggest potential palliatives. This exercise is important as one must avoid replicating these limitations in any proposed, more expansive, pathology diagnosing infrastructure. Second, I draw out the core utility of potential non-monistic, non-neo-Idealist recognition accounts. It is worth ascertaining precisely what, if anything, recognition theory has to offer a rejuvenated Critical Theory. Third, borne out of this preceding discussion, I present a radically reconfigured recognition framing, capturing the insights, while cautious of the many weaknesses of, recognition theory.

In this third section, I argue that an analysis of recognition claims can potentially become part of a more inclusive pathology diagnosing analysis, not due to the alleged innate emancipatory potential of the 'recognition moment' (Honneth, 1995), but, on the contrary, precisely because such claims for recognition evince the workings of constitutive power while retaining a focus on the subject (Thompson, 2016; 2019). In my suggested reconfiguration, what to the contemporary recognition approach is a foundational weakness, namely that recognition claims are not immune to the effects of social-structural power (McNay, 2008), can become, in a reoriented account, a core asset. Analysing recognition claims could become a means for engaging with the impact of social-structures and their constitutive power upon the social subject. A reworked recognition approach can thus help identify pathological demands *for* recognition, rather than to expose solely pathological denials *of* recognition (Canivez, 2011).

Through this proposed reformulation of recognition theory both pathological claims for recognition, and some of the pathological logics which produce them, can be identified. However, echoing Thompson, I hold that such 'constitutive logics' exist beyond the scope of the recognition register (Thompson, 2016; 2019). In my suggested approach, looking at recognition claims is helpful in that it offers *an entry point* to engaging with these alternate, deeper structural dynamics, without viewing these logics as primarily intersubjective. Thus, while the reformulation of recognition I advance here engages with subjects' purported experience of misrecognition, the social theorist must immediately draw on other non-recognition frameworks to further their analyses. My reframing thus utilises recognition theory for two purposes: a) to draw out pathological demands for recognition, and b) to function as an entry point to identify the deeper social pathologies which produce these expectations.

Through the presentation of this reconfigured recognition framework, this chapter offers a way in which recognition theory can potentially be utilised as part of a broader, non-exclusionary, pathology diagnosing endeavour, while remaining aware of the serious limitations of the Honnethian paradigm. This chapter is also presented as a means of bridging otherwise siloed literatures. Contemporary recognition theorists have been loathed to accept the limitations of their approach and have thus failed to meliorate potent criticisms levelled at their theoretical foundations (Chapter Three). This chapter seeks to take seriously such concerns and considers possibilities for radically reorienting the recognition approach, while remaining committed to a 'undomesticated' Critical Theory.

The pitfalls to avoid

it is worth retracing the core limitations of mainstream recognition approaches to avoid replicating these weaknesses in a broader pathology diagnosing infrastructure. In this section I argue that many of the core principles of contemporary recognition approaches are problematic and must be discarded.

Current recognition approaches:

1. are damagingly, and unnecessarily exclusionary,

2. have developed a restrictive cognitive framing,

3. afford an unjustifiable ontological primacy to the intersubjective moment,

4. are neo-Idealist in that they present recognition relationships as harbouring a unique, intrinsic emancipatory potential, and,

5. contend that all aspects of the social world can be grasped through a recognition optic.

The Exclusionary Nature of the Recognition Paradigm

As the preceding three chapters have stressed (Chapters Four to Six), a key weakness of dominant recognition theoretical approaches is that they exclude other, more potent means of engaging with social pathologies. Fraser submitted as early as 2001 that the central weakness of dominant recognition approaches is that they are absolutely 'convinced that the terms of recognition must represent the *unified* framework for [the Critical Theoretical] … project' (Fraser and Honneth, 2001: 113, my italics). From such an exclusionary recognition optic, even 'distributional injustices must be understood as the institutional expression of … unjustified relations of recognition (Fraser and Honneth, 2001: 114). Yet, as my engagements with Rousseau, Hegel and Fromm have demonstrated, the distribution of social resources is much more complex than this position allows. Dominant recognition approaches fail to acknowledge that there any many forms of social pathology which cannot be captured by the recognition optic, while there are more which, while partially-intelligible to recognition frameworks,[133] are more cogently and intuitively theorised through other social-theoretical infrastructure. I have justified this point at length in Chapters Four to Six. As argued in these chapters, there are potent alternate social theoretical frameworks to engage with species of social pathology which are

---

[133] For instance, Schaub and Odigbo (2019) have recently attempted to present a taxonomy of the pathologies in the economic sphere solely utilising the recognition approach. Even if this endeavour was entirely successful (I argue elsewhere it was not) they could surely have made a more intuitive analysis of the pathologies of the economic realm utilising a non-recognition derived approach.

completely incompatible with, and invisible to, recognition-derived approaches (Chapters Four to Six).

It is essential that in their inclusion of recognition insights as part of a broader pathology diagnosing endeavour, Critical Theorists do not view society solely, or primarily, as the social manifestation of recognition relationships (Fraser and Honneth, 2001; McNay, 2008; Thompson, 2016). Yet, to date, many theorists maintain a staunch fidelity to a strictly recognition-derived approach, which serves to exclude all other modes of engagement with social pathologies through the needlessly restrictive definition advanced for 'social pathology'.[134] In contrast, for Critical Theorists to benefit from the breadth of efficacious framings of social pathology available, it is essential for recognition theorists to surrender the claim to be able to comprehend the social totality through the recognition optic (Fraser and Honneth, 2001). The social world is much more than an interconnected web of recognition relationships, there are important hierarchies that impact subjects beyond the intersubjective register (Thompson, 2019). This realisation is essential for social theorists to begin to understand the social realities which produce pathological demands for, and denials of, recognition.

The Recognition-Cognitive Turn

The last decade has witnessed the ascendancy of a recognition-cognitive framing of social pathology (Chapter Three). While the antecedent recognition approach was restrictive insofar as it viewed the entirety of the social world solely through a recognition optic, the recognition-cognitive perspective furthers this exclusionary tendency. As expressed in Chapter Three, an influential article by Zurn suggested that social pathologies should be defined as 'second order disconnects', as failures of the social subject to realise the emancipatory potential of mutual recognition relationships (Zurn, 2011: 345). Echoing Freyenhagen (2015), I commented how such an approach is unacceptable from multiple perspectives (Chapter Three). The recognition-cognitive turn in social pathology scholarship must, therefore, be reconsidered. Such an approach is too restrictive not merely in its failure to engage with various types of problematic recognition relationships due to its narrow cognitivism (Freyenhagen, 2015; Laitinen, 2015), but more broadly in its inability to engage with the multiple framings of social pathology which are inaccessible to intersubjective approaches (as discussed above).

---

[134] Schaub and Odigbo's paper (mentioned in footnote 1, above) epitomises this position.

The Purported Ontological Primacy of Recognition

As established in Chapter Two, a central criticism levelled at recognition theoretical approaches is of the ontological primacy afforded to the intersubjective moment (McNay, 2008; Thompson, 2016). As a result of the foundational nature accorded to the recognition dyad, all other social realities are recast as 'post hoc effect(s)' (McNay, 2008: 47). Recognition-theoretical accounts which hold this ontological commitment are unable to engage with 'a socio-structural account of power' existing beyond, or antecedent to, recognition relations (McNay, 2008: 47-48). Such an approach is not only philosophically untenable considering the presence of broader and antecedent social hierarchies (Thompson, 2019), but, again, serves to further exclude alternate framings of social pathology which are held to be 'exogenous factor(s) that comes to operate *post hoc* upon the recognition dynamic' (McNay, 2008: 72). It is imperative to move beyond any claims to the ontological primacy of the recognition moment. if recognition insights are to serve a productive role as part of a philosophically justifiable broader pathology diagnosing endeavour.

Emancipatory Potential

A central facet of Honnethian recognition theory is the claim that the intersubjective moment has unique emancipatory potential (Honneth, 1995; Laitinen, Särkelä, and Ikäheimo, 2015). It is essential that such claims are dispensed with (Chapter Two). Recall that for recognition theorists, society is nothing more than 'extrapolations of psychic dynamics' (McNay, 2008: 138). As established above, with the ontological primacy placed on the recognition moment, recognition theorists posit a 'unidirectional causal dynamic' between the cognitive-intersubjective and the social (McNay, 2008: 138). Emancipation thus necessitates interventions within the recognition order. As Thompson (2016; 2019) and McNay (2008) have argued, such claims are built upon philosophically unjustifiable foundations. For Thompson such purported emancipation-through-recognition is irredeemably neo-Idealist in that it ascribes to the subject cognitive capacities which are impervious to social power (Thompson, 2016). Yet, recognition is not the originary site of social life; there are structures and hierarchies antecedent to, and impacting upon, subjectivation (Thompson, 2016: 5-12; 2019). To incorporate the positive insights of recognition theory as part of a multilateral Critical Theory one must commence by renouncing the claim that the recognition dyad has unique, emancipatory potential. The cognitive and intersubjective capacities of the subject must be understood as impacted upon by social structural forces which transcend the intersubjective register.

The Untargeted Application of 'Recognition' to all Social Domains

A constant theme in the foregoing discussion is the damaging trend within contemporary social theory to view all aspects of the social world through the recognition lens. In a recent paper in the *European Journal of Social Theory*, Schaub and Odigbo (2019) epitomise this tendency. They advance a 'complete typology' of the pathologies of the economic sphere utilising the recognition approach. For Schaub and Odigbo, the reliance of around a million people in the UK on foodbanks is evidence of 'consumptive need misrecognition'. Such a commitment to the recognition approach seems absurd because, as Fraser has articulately argued, 'not all maldistribution is a by-product of misrecognition' (Fraser and Honneth, 2001: 35). Indeed, the increasing need for the precariat to turn to foodbanks, pay-day lenders and support from family and friends, can be best understood as a direct result of the shifting 'balance of power between labor and capital' (Fraser and Honneth, 2001: 215) due to political-economic dynamics which are once-removed from the intersubjective register. Further, Schaub and Odigbo's recognition-derived submission may be read as serving to occlude the political culpability of the actors who furthered the 'Austerity' agenda (Coulthard, 2014; Siddique, 2018). As has been established in the previous chapters, the logics and dynamics Fraser refers to are inaccessible to a restrictive recognition approach. The solution, again, seems immediately apparent. Where there is a plethora of alternate, non-recognition factors at work, adopting a primarily recognition optic is extremely counter-productive. Thus, for the insights of recognition theory to be of use to a broader, social pathology diagnosing project, it is essential that the recognition register is turned to when investigating pathological status differentials, or where a recognition approach can offer a useful entry point for a broader, polycentric enquiry.

The utility to be harnessed

While the limitations of the dominant recognition paradigm are substantial, I have offered plausible routes through which these can be mitigated. True, my engagement serves to radically reorient, and in some ways to neuter, the recognition paradigm. This may prove unacceptable to many of the committed recognition theorists who staunchly utilise the perspective regardless of the increasingly publicised accounts of its limitations.[135] That stated, while the preceding discussion serves to negate many of the more radical claims of recognition theory, I argue that the following three features of the approach are of utility and can be incorporated as part of a

---

[135] As I state in an introductory article to a special edition of *The European Journal of Social Theory*, the scholarly debate surrounding the utility of the recognition paradigm has become calcified and hotly contested. There would be a real utility for social theory more broadly if recognition theorists were to seriously engage with the arguments presented against their approach and enter into productive dialogue.

broader pathology diagnosing project. I submit that the central strengths of the recognition approaches are:

1. the empirically agreed need for recognition, and how this awareness has been mobilised as a foundation for undergirding normative theory,
2. their ability to engage with the affective experiences of social subjects, and,
3. the ability to provide an entry point for broader social critique which centres the subject.

The empirically agreed need for recognition

Honneth has been consistent in pointing to the empirical evidence supporting the need for intersubjective recognition (Honneth, 1995).[136] Honneth's ground-breaking book *The Struggle for Recognition* was thus able to present a 'social theory with normative content' in 'conditions of post-metaphysical thinking' (Honneth, 1995: 1) in which normative claims can be derived from a weak formal anthropology: that is, in the biological need for recognition. Such analysis built upon Taylor's successful popularisation of the language of 'recognition', but invested it further with empirical, scientific insights (Taylor, 1994). Through a turn to Winnicott (1965, 1971) and Stern (1985), recognition-theorists have been able to argue, empirically, that recognition is important for the maintenance of a healthy self-relation throughout the entirety of the life-course.

Such an approach has two key characteristics which can be productively incorporated into a broader, pathology diagnosing endeavour. The first is immediately apparent: there is clearly a need to engage with recognition where appropriate, and one must likewise accept that when the subject seeks recognition from irrational sources they are likely to encounter developmental and psychological problems.[137] Further, the irrational denial of recognition is, as recognition theorists suggest, a social pathology. Social norms and values which serve to systematically denigrate subjects, such that they are irrationally denied respect, love and esteem are thus, undeniably, one species of social pathology (Hirvonen, 2015).

---

[136] It is interesting that Honneth turns repeatedly to Donald Winnicott (1965, 1971) to further this point (Honneth, 1995: 98-106), yet only mentions the work of Daniel Stern fleetingly (Honneth, 1995: 97). Stern's *The Interpersonal World of the Infant* (1985) would appear, *prima facie*, to have been a more intuitive port of call.

[137] Yet a consideration which has not been thoroughly interrogated in the literature more broadly is the need to place the demands for recognition of a 'confused' or 'anomic' subject, or a subject socialised in a world with classed, raced and gendered power gradients, relative to the requirements for a rational society more broadly. This may require denying recognition claims from many subjects who will initially suffer as a result. How this should be managed while acknowledging that racist/sexist/classed demands for esteem are a product of social processes more broadly, requires further discussion.

Yet, contra to leading recognition theoretical approaches, it proves hard to determine when claims of misrecognition are, and are not, justified (Canivez, 2011). As Critical Theorists stress, both the dominant, irrational forms of social organisation, and the ideologically imbued, limited forms of consciousness they sustain, serve to impede the subject's capacity to provide an unmediated, 'objective' account and analysis of their lived experiences. While pathologies of recognition clearly do exist, and there is empirical evidence pointing towards the harm denied recognition can precipitate (Honneth, 1995), because of the complexity and irrationality of the social world it is less clear precisely what the theorist can do with this knowledge. Ultimately this central recognition theoretical insight is less productive that one might immediately be inclined to think. Extending my previous arguments, despite the empirical evidence pointing to the need for love, respect and esteem in, and from, recognition relationships, it does not follow that all pathologies are, in the final instance, derivative of problematic recognition relationships. Neither does it inevitably follow that the harms of denied recognition are always best theorised through an exclusively recognition paradigm.

Further still, and perhaps most problematic for ardent recognition theorists, just because a subject is harmed by not being recognised in a certain way does not mean that they necessarily merit such recognition. A racist may genuinely feel aggrieved and injured when people of colour fail to show them significant respect, and the racist may suffer a genuine psychic injury as a result of the disconnect between his demand for recognition and his experience of its denial (see footnote 5). In Honnethian terms, the esteem a subject may enjoy from the subservience of others may form of critical aspect of their healthy self-relation. Yet it is absurd to argue that the bigot is entitled to recognition as racially superior because it aids their healthy relation-to-self.[138] It is thus much harder to action a research programme that is *philosophically justifiable* based on the analysis of subject's claims to denied recognition than one might think.[139] As I shall argue in the following section, Critical Theorists might productively commence their analysis by examining a subject's claims of denied recognition, but such testimony alone is of limited use. Given that recognition relationships occur within a broader social world, shaped by social-

---

[138] Consider the final scene of the 1957 Henry Fonda film, *12 Angry Men*. 'Juror 3', an older white man, initially refuses to acknowledge the possibility of the defendant being innocent. The patient argumentation from Fonda ('Juror 8') gradually leads to all but Juror 3 accepting the likelihood of the defendant's innocence. When it becomes clear that Juror 3's opinion, laced with prejudices and ageist, classist bigotry, is not being respected by the other jurors, he breaks down in tears. The denial of esteem to subject's can cause a rupture of their self-image, the disconnect between their expectations for, and experiences of, (mis-)recognition marking a true breach for the individual's self-relation.

[139] Developing footnote 5 (above): This is not to state that recognition has not been productively utilised in the numerous instances eluded to in this paper. The point here, however, is that the precise theoretical framework may not present the optimum means of engaging with the constitutive powers that shape social subjects, and which thus impact greatly on their demands for recognition.

structural powers and hierarchies, such claims will always need to be engaged with relative to a broader analysis of constitutive power (Thompson, 2016; 2019). This necessitates moving beyond the intersubjective register (Thompson, 2016; 2019). Such considerations rarely feature in the dominant recognition approaches (Thompson, 2016: Chapter One-Three).

Thus, a measured conclusion must be drawn here: recognition theorists have a valid insight insofar as the denial of recognition can cause subjects empirically verifiable harm. The presence of social logics which serve to *irrationally* deny subjects esteem, love and respect are therefore pathological. However, such a realisation needs to be measured, and soundly incorporated within the plethora of alternate social maladies which beset the social world. One cannot examine such social-structural logics solely through an engagement with subjects' testimony (Canivez, 2011). As stated, the denial of recognition to a subject, while evincing a short-term harm, may in some instances produce a greater social good for the subject, and a longer term good for the broader society. The conclusions which can be legitimately drawn here is that recognition relationships merit analysis, and that subject's claims of denied recognition can provide an important entry point to social critique. However, such analysis must always be measured and held as part of a broader polycentric pathology diagnosing framework.

Second, emerging from the empirical work pointing to the need for recognition, there are advantages to the turn to a weak formal anthropology as the basis for conducting critical social theory. I have previously outlined the merits of such an approach, which has been best advanced by Honneth's recognition theory (Chapter One). Yet, it must be stated that while a weak formal anthropology has perhaps been best incorporated in critical social theory through Honneth's recognition approach, there is no essential need for such a 'normative fix' to occur through recognition. Indeed, Fromm's 'normative humanism' (Chapter Six) could equally justifiably serve to provide such a framing (Thompson A 2009; Thompson M J, 2014). The empirically verifiable need for recognition thus brings two further beneficial insights for broader pathology diagnosing social theory: the utility of basing critical social theory with normative content in a weak formal anthropology, and the need to engage, as part of a broader project, with pathologies of recognition.

Means of critically engaging with the subject's affective experience

Recognition theoretical approaches offer an intuitive way to engage with a truly immanent aspect of the social world: subjects' lived reality of suffering and disrespect. The recognition approach allows the researcher to directly engage with the subject's sense of hurt, or denied esteem, across contexts. It has thus been utilised to further social research across the breadth of the social word, from elder care (Niemi, 2015) to music-schools (Elmgren, 2015), even into contemporary populist movements (Hirvonen and Pennanen, 2019). This adaptability is achieved while constantly retaining the focus on the individual's psychological experience. This ability to engage with the subject's lived reality is undeniably central to the popularity of the recognition paradigm. A broader social pathology diagnosing approach must learn from recognition theorists on the importance of being able to engage with the subject's affective experiences, as and when appropriate.

That stated, one must caution against blindly centring the purportedly injured subject, divining "social truths" from their affective responses to their perceived denied recognition. Harding's 'standpoint theory', for instance, falls into the trap of privileging the truth content of marginalised subjects, viewing their narratives as inherently harbouring a 'strong objectivity' (Harding, 2004). For Harding, the voices of subaltern subjects are of greater value to the social theorist than the presentations of 'non-oppressed' social actors, as the 'outsider-within' experience produces 'bicultural' knowledge. In addition to the well-trodden critiques of essentialism which have dogged Harding's work (Harraway, 1988; Code, 2008), one must also caution the multiple problems with determining who really is misrecognised, who really is the marginalised subject. Further, there are disconnects between the lived realities of precarious subjects (people of colour, for example) and their narratives of disrespect and misrecognition. Embodiment, subjecthood, and critical cognition do not exist in a coherent, predetermined unity or symmetry. Currently in the UK, for example, the Home Secretary, Sajid Javid, a second-generation immigrant, is responsible for enforcing a racist immigration policy which separates migrant families, causing devastating consequences (Younge, 2018). The ability to engage with subjects' affective realities has only served to bolster the popularity of the recognition paradigm among social researchers, however, as argued, engagement with affective experiences, as a theoretical and research focus, must not precipitate uncritically granting epistemic privilege to the accounts of those who purport misrecognition.

A means to further social theory centring, but not limited to, the subject

Perhaps the most useful aspect of a recognition derived approach for Critical Theory is that it enables the social subject to be centred as a springboard from which to conduct deeper, structural analysis. While above I commented on the utility of recognition accounts engaging with the subject's affective experiences, this broader benefit can too easily be overlooked. While Honnethian recognition theorists problematically consider that the entirety of the social world can be adequately theorised as a 'recognition network' (Fraser and Honneth, 2001), their position has one clear benefit: it locates the individual's experience (of denied recognition) relative to broader social-structural logics (the logics and structures of a broader recognition network). The immediacy with which such an approach enables the theorist to move between the individual's affective experience and broader social logics is enviable. While I criticise the limitations of the recognition framing more broadly, the ability to shift focus between subject and social logics effortlessly is an important target to aim for in a reformulated pathology diagnosing Critical Theory.

Concluding thoughts on the utility of recognition theory

A considered recognition approach clearly harbours utility. The challenge is to engage these efficacious aspects of recognition theoretical accounts while addressing their manifold limitations. As this section has demonstrated, the key advantages of a recognition approach are the ability to engage with subjects' real-world experiences of suffering and to use this as an entry point for broader social critique. This renewed focus could, for example, help Critical Theory overcome the criticism that it is overinvested in the analysis of social-structural logics and negates, and occludes, the lived realities of social subjects (Freundlieb, 2015). In contrast, as I suggest below, one can centre the subject's experiences of misrecognition to facilitate broader social-structural analysis, and, by doing so, move beyond the recognition-register.

Incorporating recognition as part of a broader social pathology diagnosing infrastructure

From the preceding discussion it has become apparent that a radically reoriented recognition account is required for any of the recognition framing's insights to sit happily as part of a broader pathology diagnosing endeavour. In the following section I will present a possible reformulation, seeking to appropriate the useful facets of recognition theory, while negating the philosophically untenable and social-theoretically restrictive features of the Zurnian-Honnethian paradigm. I suggest that Critical Theorists might productively engage the tools provided by recognition theory as one means amongst others for conducting pathology diagnosing social critique. Where a research subject, whether explicitly or implicitly, contends they are suffering from denied recognition, it makes complete sense for the Critical Theorist to commence their analysis utilising a recognition-derived framework. I diverge from the orthodoxy, however, by suggesting that the Critical Theorist should utilise the subjects' claims of denied recognition as an entry point for probing the broader social conjecture, and, in so doing, swiftly transcend the recognition framework. My core submission here is that the subjects' purported denied recognition might productively be engaged with as testimony to the types of recognition they have been conditioned to expect by the constitutive power of their social world.

In contrast to orthodox recognition approaches, which focus on subjects' experiences of inadequate or denied recognition, I am arguing that the Critical Theorist should examine the pathological nature of irrational demands *for* recognition. Again, it is crucial to stress that I do not believe in some latent emancipatory potential lurking within a foundational dyadic relationship. In my suggested approach, the turn to the recognition register is of use only insofar as it offers an entry point to the social world, to help illuminate the mechanisms of constitutive power (Thompson, 2016). The subject's testimony of having experienced denied recognition is of use to the Critical Theorist, not because it holds a determinate truth content, but because it demonstrates the belief of the social subject. The subject feels that they have been denied recognition; that, and that alone, is a promising entry point for critical social theory and social research. It is with this central insight that the recognition register offers a useful resource as part of a broader, pathology diagnosing endeavour.

In contrast to the dominant approach which focuses on pathological denials of recognition, I following Canivez (2011), argue that it is essential that theorists realise the possibility that a subject's claimed denied recognition, while felt intensely, may be due to their own irrational expectations of love, respect or esteem. One must thus consider the pathological nature of many claims *for* recognition. Consider for instance a racist, misogynistic white male's expectations of recognition from black women. One must retain an awareness that the subject is socialised in a world impacted by logics of constitutive power which impact the subject's expectations of recognition relationships.

To give this approach more substance, imagine a second hypothetical scenario, where a sociologist is conducting research into the various social pathologies pertinent to Brexit. The researcher may engage with a subject who comments that they feel deeply disrespected by the foreign nationals living in 'their' community, who they see as failing to integrate, despite living in the same neighbourhood, or working for the same employer. The research subject may claim that they feel 'disrespected' as the foreign nationals seem 'surly', 'unsmiling' and 'fail to catch the eye' of the subject (see Burnett, 2017). While the traditional recognition perspective would be limited to engaging with this testimony as potentially demonstrating the failure of healthy recognition relationships to have developed in the more diverse community, my suggested approach would start from the subject's testimony, and use it as an entry point to consider the constitutive power relations which led to their expectations and precipitant sense of disrespect (Canivez, 2011).

In contrast to viewing the purported denial of recognition as evincing a pathological failure in the development of relations of recognition, the researcher would use the testimony gathered as an entry point to consider broader social-structural logics. The researcher could thus consider the impact of the 'hostile environment' (Grierson, 2018), the impact of neoliberal casualisation of labour (Kapoor, 2013), and the breakdown of community institutions. The examination of the social irrationality, which was commenced by the testimony of denied recognition by the research subject, has thus cascaded outwards to consider the myriad of constitutive factors which impact upon the subject's socialisation. Viewing the 'failure to catch the eye' as no longer a deficient part of a primary intersubjective dyadic relationship which should be accorded ontological primacy, but as the result of broader, social-structural processes which impact upon all social subjects, the failure of harmonious intersubjective relations is held to be symptomatic of deeper social pathologies.

In my reconfigured account, an analysis of recognition claims may function as a possible entry point to a broader, multi-pronged analysis. I reiterate that I propose that recognition might function merely as *one* entry point to the social, not the sole, nor the dominant means of commencing social research. However, where explicitly relevant, as in the case of the hypothetical example above, and when suitably extracted from the dominant Honnethian approach, it can offer a meaningful manner to commence social theory and social research. Despite the manifold failings of the Honnethian paradigm, it remains the case that there are social pathologies which can be productively engaged with through the recognition register. This reality, however, does not mean that all pathologies are recognition-derived, or that the recognition framing harbours unique critical potency (Fraser and Honneth, 2001; Thompson, 2016).

My suggested approach can be summarised in four key steps. First, where appropriate, I propose that the recognition framework can be adapted and adopted as one possible entry point to the social world (amongst various others). Second, I suggest that the researcher must adopt a 'value neutral' engagement relative to recognition claims: they must jettison any notion that there lies some latent emancipatory potential lurking in the subject's experiences of some purportedly 'primal' intersubjective dyad. The presumption that denied recognition is the attendant social pathology needs to be rejected. Third, the Critical Theorist then engages with the subject's affective resonances to determine how and why they feel mis/un-recognised. The given responses are utilised to help draw out the workings and machinations of constitutive power upon the subject. Fourth, through an analysis of the position of the subject, relative to the power gradients presented through an analysis of the dynamics of constitutive power and the broader social-structural realities, the theorist may comment on the rationality, or irrationality, of the subject's claim *for* recognition.

By viewing the subject's claimed denied recognition relative to the workings of broader social-structural logics, the Critical Theorist comments not on the presence (or absence) of pathologically denied recognition, but on the rationality of the subject's claim *for* recognition. The objective which is centred in my alternate approach to recognition is the development of analyses which help identify broader social-structural pathologies which lead to the development of irrational claims for recognition.

How Such an Approach Avoids the Pitfalls of Contemporary Recognition Framings

My suggested approach for harnessing the utility of the recognition approach avoids the pitfalls of neo-Idealism as it focuses on the content of the recognition claims themselves, offering a route to investigate constitutive power relations. Neither the intersubjective moment, nor the epistemic capacity of the 'injured' subject are granted ontological or epistemic primacy or privilege. In direct contrast to dominant approaches to recognition theory, in my proposed reframing the subject's sense of denied recognition is held to be impacted by broader social-structural logics.

As stressed, my proposed approach does not echo the exclusionary tendencies of the dominant recognition-cognitive, or other recognition-theoretical framework(s). As presented throughout, I consider that this approach offers one possible route, but one possible route amongst many, for engaging with social pathologies. Perhaps more importantly, I do not argue, even when utilising the recognition framework, that the pathological aspect of society is to be located within the intersubjective dyad. In my presentation there is no antecedent 'failure' of recognition, from which a pathological society is projected. In contrast, the subject's sense of denied recognition is presented as a means of engaging with irrational social logics more broadly. Such irrational social developments are best framed through the multiple species of social pathology which have been outlined through Chapters Four-Six. There is thus always a need to engage with multiple species of social pathology beyond recognition, even though, in certain instances, a recognition approach can be of great utility.

As discussed, there has been a growing tendency to present all social pathologies as projections of irrational recognition relationships (Harris, 2019). My engagement with recognition, as advanced here, would function solely to allow critical theorists the benefit of the theoretical infrastructure where it is apposite, but would have no bearing on pathological social dynamics where the intersubjective dimension is not a primary concern.

How Such an Approach Harnesses the Potential of the Recognition Optic

While I support Fraser's assertion that there are many areas of social life which have 'little to do with recognition' (Fraser and Honneth, 2001: 35), she herself states (Fraser and Honneth, 2001: 2-5), there are also occasions where a cautious recognition theoretical approach could be very useful to the Critical Theorist, if the foundational weaknesses of the Honnethian account could be vitiated. The reformulation of recognition presented above follows traditional recognition approaches insofar as it commences the analysis of the social world through initially centring the subject's sense of disrespect, or misrecognition. The approached championed here retains this ability to engage with the affective aspect of the subject's lived reality without unduly privileging the content of the subject's testimony.

While my reformulation here does not hold recognition relationships to be the primal, foundational core of the social order, it retains an awareness that irrational recognition relationships need to be incorporated in a broader pathology diagnosing infrastructure. By locating a subject's claims for recognition within the broader social-structural reality, the theorist may determine whether the subject's claim for recognition is itself irrational.

My proposed reconfiguration of recognition rests on the social researcher placing the subject's claimed experience of misrecognition within the broader social world. It is only when subjects' purported claims of denied recognition are placed relative to the broader forms of constitutive power that the rationality of the recognition relationship as a whole can be analysed. What is distinct about my approach is that the social researcher would arrive at such a conclusion, not on the basis of the testimony of the 'misrecognised', or by examining the broader psychological impact of the intersubjective dyad, but by examining the constitutive power that 'pulse(s) beneath the surface' of social action' (Thompson, 2016: 7).

Conclusion

As this thesis argues throughout, the dominant recognition-derived approaches for engaging with the social world are deeply problematic. This Honnethian paradigm is needlessly exclusionary and philosophically and social theoretically unjustifiable. That stated, as this chapter argues, a radically reworked recognition optic could play a partial role as part of a broader 'multilateral' Critical Theoretical endeavour (Fraser and Honneth, 2001: 209). For this to be possible, however, several of the central claims of the recognition approach would need to be dismissed. This chapter thus started by briefly retracing the central limitations of the dominant recognition approach, and provided possible solutions for their overcoming. The second part of the chapter then presented the primary merits of the recognition approach. With this groundwork completed, I was able to offer my suggested reformulated recognition approach, which I propose could play a small part in a broader theoretical infrastructure for engaging with social pathologies.

Echoing Fraser, I 'object in principle to *any* proposal to ground a normative framework on one privileged set of experiences' (Fraser and Honneth, 2001: 205 – my italics). My proposed reformulation of recognition did not confer an epistemic or ontological primacy to either the recognition moment, or to the subject's post-hoc reflections on their affective responses to their intersubjective relationships. Rather, I suggested that recognition could play an important role in a broader pathology diagnosing endeavour as an entry point to the social world which illuminates the workings of constitutive power and the dynamics of social-structures.

Far from placing 'all its eggs in one basket' (Fraser and Honneth, 2001: 205), this reconfigured approach to recognition would utilise aspects of the recognition register, where appropriate, as part of a broader pathology diagnosing exercise. Engaging with subjects' claims for recognition can be a useful starting point for theorists seeking to diagnose social pathologies as it offers an immediate presentation of the demands and expectations of the social subject and it offers a ready means of engaging with affective experience. My reason for engaging with recognition claims is thus highly divergent from the dominant orthodoxy. In my approach there is no presumption that the irrationality of the social world stems from denied recognition. In contrast, this chapter has argued that a reconfigured recognition framework can play a role in a broader social pathology diagnosing endeavour insofar as it can help identify the pathological nature of many subjects' demands *for* recognition, and it can offer an entry point to analyse pathological social structural realities which transcend the recognition register.

162

Conclusion

Social Pathology Diagnosis and the Future of Critical Theory

This conclusion is divided into three sections. First, I comment on how a rejuvenated pathology diagnosing social theory can help inform future social research. Second, I argue for the importance of a polycentric pathology diagnosing approach for renewing the radicalism of the broader Critical Theoretical project. Third, I abstract the social-theoretical submission at the core of the thesis, which is presented as a distinctive and timely intervention in a contested literature.

Social Pathology Diagnosis and Social Research

As Chapter Six of this thesis drew out, one of the central research questions for the Frankfurt School was 'how can people accept the brutalities of the present as an acceptable normality?' (Fromm, 2010). Expressed more politically, first-generation Critical Theorists sought to answer: 'Why isn't there revolutionary social change?' (Bronner, 2002, 2011; Held, 2013; Jeffries, 2017). In response, they discovered various social pathologies which furthered subjects' susceptibility to reactionary, even fascist, dispositions (Adorno, Frenkel-Brunswik, Levinson and Sanford, 1950; Fromm, 1963, 2010). For Adorno and Fromm, *inter alia*, the practice of Critical Theory itself, the very diagnosis of social pathologies, marked an important part in the reclamation of critical subjectivity. Critical Theory is how consciousness fights back (Jay, 2016). However, Critical Theory, from its inception, focused equally on researching the objective contradictions operating within social organisations and structures, in addition to exploring the ideological impediments to critical consciousness (Strydom, 2011). In the first section of this conclusion, I thus draw out the importance of undergirding social research with a multifaceted pathology diagnosing social theory, both for examining the impeded critical capacity of the individual *and* for investigating the pathologies of the objective social world (Delanty, 2011).

For Hoy and McCarthy (1994), it is essential that the theoretical foundations provided by Critical Theorists can animate research projects on both concerns. It is only through the excoriating analysis of both objective societal irrationalities, and of the shared cognitive impairments which occlude them from popular consciousness, that Critical Theory can truly make its presence felt as a political force (Bronner, 2011; Delanty, 2011). It is thus important to establish how and why my proposed 'multilateral and polycentric' pathology diagnosing social theory can provide a robust foundation for social research (Fraser and Honneth, 2001: 209).

Throughout this thesis, numerous displaced framings of social pathology have been critically discussed, all of which, I have argued, are of utility for social *theory*. Before I demonstrate how and why these framings can also help facilitate social *research*, I briefly recount the multiple efficacious framings of social pathology excavated throughout this thesis.

The Multiple Framings of Social Pathology

Chapters Four to Six drew out various framings of social pathology which are substantially excluded by the dominant recognition paradigm. While this was admittedly a partial and incomplete project (there are a multitude of alternate framings of social pathology), this engagement satisfied two objectives. First, it drew out the limited scope of the dominant recognition-derived approach to engaging with social pathologies. Second, it demonstrated the critical utility harboured by neglected framings of social pathology.

In the analysis of Rousseau (Chapter Four), five distinct framings of social pathology were drawn out:

f)   self-perpetuating negative dynamics,

g)   unstructured dependency,

h)   cultural pathology,

i)   the colonisation of one social sphere by the logic of another, and

j)   multiple layers of recognition pathology.

Developing Neuhouser's argument (2012), I submitted that these framings provide an apposite means for engaging with the irrationalities manifest in today's social world as they enable Critical Theorists to delve 'deeper' than liberal social critique and thus to move beyond the dominant concerns of justice and legitimacy.

The discussion on 'pathologies of reason' (Chapter Five), drew out the utility of diagnosing discrepancies[140] between the dominant organisational logics of the objective social world and the more rational potential latent within them (Honneth, 2007b: 21). The diagnosis of such 'pathologies of reason' offers an important framework for social research, as it brings forth Critical Theory's uniquely progressive methodology: immanent-transcendence. For Strydom, it is this future-oriented nature of Critical Theory, derived from this methodological commitment, which distinguishes Critical Theoretical social research from other research programmes (Strydom, 2011: 9).[141] Such a focus can be carried out through a diagnosis of social pathologies of reason, and can thus propel social research in its uniquely future-oriented direction.

---

[140] Perhaps 'lags' is a more apposite term.

[141] As Strydom draws out, neither empiricism not rationalism nor idealism are fundamentally annexed to a 'forward-looking' social philosophy or social project (Strydom, 2011: 9-11). The focus on exploring potentialities for immanent-transcendence thus marks Critical Theory as methodologically unique in its future orientation.

Chapter Six, the discussion of Fromm's (1963, 1979, 2010, *inter alia*) scholarship, drew out three key components of a society evincing 'pathological normalcy'. These are: a) an analysis of the social world as incommensurable with the demands of 'normative humanism'; b) where subjects fail to realise this due to 'socially patterned defects', and c) where such a pathological state is reinforced as the norm through the process of 'consensual validation'. Fromm's underappreciated theoretical infrastructure illuminates important concerns for social theorists which remain invisible to the dominant recognition-derived paradigm.

Chapter Seven, my proposed reconfiguration of the recognition framework, also presented considerations for social research. In contrast to engaging predominantly with the intersubjective moment at the centre of a subject's purported 'denied recognition' (Honneth, 1995), I suggested that social researchers might profit from focusing on the deeper, non-recognitive pathologies present within society, manifest in subjects' often-irrational demands *for* recognition.

As Turner argues, for Critical Theory to offer any significant prospect of aiding material praxis it is essential that it conducts social research built upon solid social theoretical foundations (Turner, 2009: 4-6). Of course, this is not to suggest that social theory without an attendant social research programme is impotent. Adorno would have viewed any such suggestion as epitomising the extractive, instrumentalising, and positivistic traits of a society riven by capitalist domination, a typical 'compromise with "the given"' (Durkin, 2019: 106). Rather, Turner's (2009) submission, following Horkheimer (1975), is that an optimal Critical Theory requires the seamless interplay of social theory and social research. The social-theoretical project at the core of this thesis hopes to contribute to such an interdisciplinary infrastructure.

Having outlined the core social-theoretical insights for social research presented in this thesis, I will now demonstrate how they can be deployed by way of the example of a pressing concern for social research: global warming.

A Potential Area for Application

The current social order is rich in pathologies, several of which are potentially existential in nature (Laitinen, 2015). Human-made global warming is perhaps the most obvious threat which endangers 'the prospects of the continuity of human life' (Chernilo, 2017: 44). In this section, I suggest that social research predicated on a pathology diagnosing theoretical infrastructure may provide new insights on this pressing concern. However, I stress that social researchers might productively engage the pathology diagnosing register to interrogate a wider range of social problems.

There is an intuitive allure to engaging with the logics and realities perpetuating global warming through the framings of social pathology (Neuhouser, 2012; Boyd, 2013). Social research could productively draw out the presence of multiple social pathologies on this pressing topic, and, through such research, might greatly heighten our understanding of the challenges and problems facing those who seek a more sustainable relationship with the global ecology. Returning to my analysis of Rousseau, social researchers could interrogate the self-perpetuating negative dynamics which exist in the political economy inhibiting moves to zero-growth (Malm, 2016; Monbiot, 2017). Equally, there is a mass of smaller scale, everyday lifestyle choices, that evince such a dynamic. Perhaps the most studied, and observably manifest example of such a dynamic, centres the increase in the popularity of air conditioning units in South Asia and North America (Pierre-Louis, 2018). Air conditioning units are in increasing demand due to increasing global temperatures. At first glance, it seems an example where the capitalist market produces and distributes a commodity of use and value to the community. However, upon closer examination, it is immediately apparent that a pathological dynamic is at work, both in the short and long-term. Air conditioning units operate by pumping hot air outside, into the street. As a result, the more residencies install air-con, the hotter the conurbation gets (Brownstone, 2014). This is in the immediate, short term. More substantially, the electricity required to operate the air-con units is still, overwhelmingly, produced by burning fossil-fuels. There is a thus a classic dynamic of negative infinity in operation: the hotter it gets the more people need air-con, the more people install air-con, the hotter it gets, *ad infinitum*. Such a social problem is best framed, and engaged with, through the rubric of social pathology.

Equally, there are various forms of cultural pathology which serve to denigrate humankind's relationship to, and dependence on, nature (Naess, 2008). The Western capitalist engagement with the broader ecology, for instance, is culturally worlds apart from a hypostatised Buddhist approach to nature (Schumacher, 1973). Neoliberal capitalism is predicated on the maintenance of unstructured relations of dependency between the human and the natural world which are unsustainable (Naess, 1989). The natural realm is conceptualised as a 'sink', an 'externality' to social production: this furthers exploitative logics which will ultimately be self-defeating due to inevitable resource scarcity (Schumacher, 1973).

There are clear pathologies of reason existing when one considers the logics which precipitate and perpetuate climate change. Contemporary society is not ignorant to the social contradictions which further global warming (Kunstler, 2012); as Strydom's recent work has drawn out, there is a 'mathematical-philosophical tradition' attuned to the importance of understanding limit constructs (Strydom, 2017: 793). Yet growth-based economics is predicated on the possibility of infinite expansion in an admittedly finite system (Bookchin, 1962; Daly, 1996).[142] There is a clear pathology of reason here, a contradiction within the immanent, which, when researched from a left-Hegelian pathologies of reason perspective, points directly towards its own sublation [Aufheben] in forms of zero-growth or alternate-growth paradigms (Borchers, 2006). The specifics of such dynamics urgently require social research (Dawson, 2019),[143] and the pathologies of reason paradigm is of utility for such an endeavour.[144]

Social researchers might productively consider the recognition pathologies which further exploitative, extractive relations towards the environment. While not adopting the terminology of 'pathology', Latour (1999) has already moved in this direction with his work on 'spokespeople' and 'actants' which draws on the broader ecological tradition (Stone, 1973). In contrast to the Honnethian paradigm's impotence on this consideration due to its foundations in intersubjectivity, my suggested approach commences with the subject's claims and attitudes in their interaction with the other, regardless of whether they constitute a subject. Those who engage in anthropocentric activities can be asked: 'What do you think about the environment?' or 'Do you feel any obligation to the broader ecosystem?' The responses can form part of a broader project of interrogating the social structures which produce subjects with explicitly anthropocentric politics.

Further, one can research both the obstacles impeding subjects' awareness of objectively pathological social dynamics and the deeper pathological normalcy which serves to foster socio-political inaction (Boyd, 2013). The simultaneous awareness of the objective reality of global warming, when viewed together with sustained political inaction suggests that the contemporary juncture has developed the characteristics of a pathological normalcy (Chapter Six). Consider how, for example, there are a great number of academics who accept global warming as an existential threat, yet continue to fly to foreign countries on holiday, drive diesels and eat steaks. I fall into this category myself. Drawing on Fromm, the public at large are lured into a pathological dynamic of mass acquiescence life continues due to the pacifying logics of pathological normalcy (Fromm, 1963, 2010). The sustained functioning of social institutions

---

[142] This text was originally published under the pseudonym Lewis Herber.
[143] While Dawson does not explicitly utilise the left-Hegelian approach, the clear focus on the contradictory state of our own awareness of crisis, and of the mathematical sophistication for modelling its likely outcomes, with such a degree of political inactivity, serves as apposite immanent critique.
[144] Lenin was famously sceptical of developing political analysis from Hegel's metaphysics stating it could 'not be *applied* in its given form ... One *must separate out* from it the logical (epistemological) nuances after purifying them from *Ideenmystik* [mystical idealism]' (Lenin: 1972: 226).

under such conditions could be fruitfully researched as evincing socially pattered cognitive defects (Fromm, 1983, 2010). Fromm would question whether those that happily conform to the continued, extractive anthropocentricism, central to the dominant neoliberal social order, are truly 'sane' (Fromm, 1963, 1979, 2010). Social research drawing on a social pathology diagnosing foundation might explicitly engage with, and expose, the dynamics which serve to impede progressive praxis. The question now becomes, how precisely is it that despite a scientifically verified wealth of knowledge which points towards the impending loss of the basic conditions necessary for life on earth within hundreds, not thousands of years, people continue largely unfazed (Klein, 2014). There are thus two distinct species of pathology here which require social research, both linking impeded cognitive capacity and broader social processes: a) the obstacles to subjects accepting the reality of human-made global warming, and b) the pathologies which impede those who have full awareness of the basic facts from making decisive changes to their lifestyles. Drawing on Fromm, one can see how a programme with a basis in diagnosing the pathologies of the normalcy can further and direct incisive social research.

This briefest of expositions has drawn out how the social pathology diagnosing approach can identify a broad array of concerns which can productively animate social research. Critical Theorists must conduct social research exploring the pathological dynamics underpinning these 'ordinary everyday social practices' (Strydom, 2011: 214). The focus on identifying social pathologies can offer a productive framework for social research into these pressing concerns.

Social Pathology Diagnosis and the Internal Politics of Contemporary Critical Theory

While this thesis primarily sits as an intervention in critical social theory, it also sits as a contribution to the broader debate igniting contemporary Critical Theory. There has been a decided shift in the core politics of the Critical Theoretical project over the past two decades. Such transitions are most clearly expressed in Thompson's *The Domestication of Critical Theory* (2016). While first-generation Critical Theorists were explicitly opposed to capitalism on the grounds that it was held to be a force of social domination inimical to critical reason, and an obstacle to a more rational society, Third and Fourth generation Critical Theorists have

> ... receded from the confrontation with the primary source of social domination and the disfiguration of human culture: capitalist market society. The theories of discourse, of recognition, or of justification that contemporary critical theory has elaborated speak more to the concerns of mainstream political philosophy than to a radical challenge to its systemic imperatives and structures of power and domination; **they play more into the very rhythms of the predominant social reality than seek any kind of social transformation**. To retrieve critical theory is to make it accountable to these structures once again (Thompson, 2016: 2 – my bold).

This shift is made further problematic, considering that:

> The dominant trends in critical theory are domesticated in that **they now seek not a confrontation with the forms of organized power that reproduce social pathologies**, but rather to articulate an academicized political philosophy sealed off from the realities that affect and deform critical subjectivity. Safe in their respective philosophical systems, they search for an emancipatory theory within the striations of everyday life (Thompson, 2016: 3 – my bold).

The Politics of Contemporary Critical Theory

While for Thompson (2016) it is Habermas who commences this retreat from the critique of capitalism, it is Honneth who most explicitly articulates the purported benefits of the capitalist order.[145] Honneth's *Freedom's Right* is particularly disturbing in its laissez-faire attitude to neoliberalism. The animus behind *Freedom's Right's* methodology of normative reconstruction is to

> examine contemporary reality in terms of its potential for fostering practices in which universal values can be realized in a superior, i.e. a more morally comprehensive and suitable fashion (Honneth, 2014b: 8).

Such an approach may *prima facie* seem similar to Critical Theory's methodology of immanent-transcendence, aiming to draw out latent higher forms of reason in the contradictions of the present, which point towards a more rational future (Strydom, 2011). However, upon closer inspection it becomes clear that this is neither Honneth's objective nor his methodology. Honneth's normative reconstruction is not a form of immanent-transcendent critique (Buchwalter, 2016). Rather, *Freedom's Right* is a political compromise with the status quo, viewing the market order as expressing, *at present*, various positive features enabling recognition (Thompson, 2016). The distinction in temporality is crucial here: for the Honneth of *Freedom's Right* these positive aspects of the capitalist order are not latent but active. *Freedom's Right* seeks to identify the *active* positives of the market order (Buchwalter, 2016). For example, Honneth draws out that implicitly, in the neoliberal market, 'subjects must recognise each other reciprocally, viewing each other as subjects' (Honneth, 2014b: 46). True, Honneth goes on to state that this form of recognition is 'egocentric' (2014b: 46), but such a caveat is hardly sufficient. Such statements of support for the emancipatory potential of social norms of capitalist society, *and explicitly of the norms intrinsic to the market order*, would simply be anathema to classical Critical Theorists such as Adorno. It is hard to deny that the Critical Theoretical project, particularly due to Honneth's influence, is experiencing an expedited change in political course. For Critical Theorists remaining attentive to the insights of first- and second-generation scholarship, Honneth's project in *Freedom's Right*, his *magnum opus* (Schaub, 2015:

---

[145] This is not to state that Honneth consistently presents such a position. Indeed, as Freyenhagen (2015) rightly comments, Honneth's *oeuvre* shows a surprising lack of political and theoretical consistency.

108), is foundationally misconceived. The reconstructive project ends up as a bizarre reactionary compromise: a non-metaphysical, post-hoc justification of the establishment. Expressed most simply, if you take the metaphysics out of Hegel's *Philosophy of Right* you are left with an infinitely weaker and more reactionary text. To a Critical Theorist more inclined to follow Thompson than Honneth, *Freedom's Right* is most illuminating not as a work of social theory, but as an indication of the domesticated state of contemporary Critical Theory.

This transition to a 'domesticated' Critical Theoretical politics is further evinced by the recent collection edited by Deutscher and Lafont (2017), *Critical Theory in Critical Times*. This text has been widely critiqued for lacking a critical political-economy and for failing to adequately interrogate the dominant sites of contemporary social domination (Thompson, 2017; Harris, 2018). While Habermas, arguably the most famous living Critical Theorist, contributed the lead paper to this collection, he was primarily concerned with problems of popular sovereignty in member states of the European Union. His presentation of the constitutional fix of 'double sovereignty' derives from the liberal tradition, not left-Hegelianism. Habermas' analysis was absent any of the concerns central to previous generations of Critical Theory: there was no trace of ideology-critique, political-economy or interdisciplinarity. To engage in a discussion on the sovereignty implications of joining the European Union without the faintest engagement with political-economy or ideology is a surreal undertaking for any social theorist. To do so in a book titled *Critical Theory in Critical Times* shows the extent to which the Critical Theoretical project has lost sight of its guiding concerns. While Habermas' paper may be interesting, in keeping with much contemporary Critical Theory it fails to offer a penetrating critique of the dominant political constellation (Harris, 2018).

Thompson's critique thus appears entirely valid: one struggles to see third- and fourth-generation Critical Theory as posing a radical critique of neoliberal capitalism and its attendant racial, gendered and anthropocentric dynamics. This thesis seeks to challenge such domesticating developments.

The Political Radicalism of a Rejuvenated Social Pathology Diagnosis

A renaissance in polycentric pathology diagnosing critique offers one route for Critical Theory to return to a direct confrontation with the manifold irrationalities of neoliberalism. This thesis explicitly supports the broader project of 'reclaiming' Critical Theory, that is returning the project to its focus on domination, political economy, and the fetters placed on critical thought by capitalist rationalities (Thompson, 2016). Shifting the focus to an open and plural engagement with social pathologies helps in this regard for three reasons.

First, the pathology diagnosing approach marks a return to the philosophical negativity of Adorno (Holloway, Matamoros and Tischler, 2009). The process of identifying social pathologies is explicitly a critique of the status quo, it is a direct attack on the *limitations* of the present conjecture (Honneth, 2000). Recent commentators have focused on the importance of Adorno's methodological embrace of negativity, how it informed both his politics and his theory (Grollios, 2017). As first-generation Critical Theorists argued, such an approach is crucial: there is no need for a positive engagement to aid progressive praxis (Adorno, 1981). For Adorno, it was philosophically and politically imperative to produce a negative critique (Adorno, 1981; O'Connor, 2004; Freyenhagen, 2013). Such an approach is in direct contradiction to the normative reconstruction which finds increasing favour in the Critical Theoretical academy today (Honneth, 2014b, Buchwalter, 2016, *inter alia*). Rather than identifying the active positives of the present, the pathology diagnosing approach returns to engaging with the contradictions and impediments to the 'actualisation' [*Verwicklichung*] of a more rational society (Bowie, 2013).

Second, a broader pathology diagnosing approach returns the analytical focus to the structural irrationalities of the political economy and their deforming impact on both consciousness and social life. Through an examination of pathological social dynamics, the manifest irrationalities of the capitalist economy are laid bare (Harvey, 2017). As I argued in Chapter Three, it was Rousseau's *Discourse on Political Economy* where such framings of social pathology were first clearly outlined. Recall that Thompson's (2016) critique of contemporary Critical Theory is that it has lost its connection to its radical forebearers and thus sits once removed from a progressive engagement with political economy.[146] Reincorporating a framing of social pathology from Rousseau's *Discourse of Political Economy* seems an apposite response to such a concern.

Third, the focus on social irrationality, integral to all framings of social pathology, and explicit in the pathologies of reason approach, serves to radically undermine the neo-Idealist paradigm, which ascribes a universal commonality, and a primacy, to the essential critical capacities of all subjects (McNay, 2008; Thompson, 2016). Engaging with the plurality of framings of social pathology advocated for in this thesis underscores how the cognitive capacities of the social subject are not constant and universal, but are multiply-mediated, impacted by historical and

---

[146] Beyond Critical Theory, in his introduction to *Marx, Capital and the Madness of Economic Reason,* Harvey has commented on the need for progressive social and political theorists to engage directly with Marx's political economy.

institutional developments.[147] Explicitly in contradiction with neo-idealism, the left-Hegelian focus on pathologies of reason insists that the social subject manifests the rational potential of the given social world. Consciousness is not a gift granted by the social body to the subject after standardised dyadic recognition relations have taken place. Rather, Marx's (1961) Copernican insight was that our capacity for critical cognition, which is a crucial antecedent for the capacity to grant recognition, is determined by the conditions of the social world, which are subject to historico-cultural variation.

With Fromm's framing of pathological normalcy the neo-Idealist tenet that the subject's cognition exists isolated from broader social-structural influences is further discredited. I thus submit that a return to a direct engagement with diagnosing the full breadth of social pathologies serves to radically destabilise the neo-Idealist paradigm due to the intrinsically 'social' nature of the social pathology framework.

While leading Critical Theorists are increasingly finding an accommodation with neoliberal capitalism, a broader framing of social pathology diagnosis, as advocated in this thesis, offers a possibility for resistance.

Restating the Central Social Theoretical Thesis

The core argument presented in this project is that the 'domesticating' unifocal recognition approach to conducting pathology diagnosing social critique must be transcended. Social theory which is limited to either the pathologies of recognition framing, or to Zurn's recognition-cognitivist approach, is philosophically unjustifiable, social-theoretically myopic, and politically impotent. In contrast, a broader, 'polycentric and multilateral' (Fraser and Honneth, 2001: 209) pathology diagnosing endeavour offers the potential for a powerful engagement with the dominant forms of institutionalised social irrationality and the equally pathological deformations of consciousness which perpetuate them. Such an analysis is impossible within the dominant Honnethian recognition framing which monopolises contemporary social pathology scholarship.

This primary submission has been developed throughout the thesis. Chapter One argued that pathology diagnosing social critique is a social-theoretically and philosophically justifiable means of conducting social criticism. The importance of 'recognition' to social theory was outlined, drawing out its distinct concerns with subjectivation, consciousness and intersubjective praxis.

---

[147] Eder (1985) takes this further, speaking of broader 'collective learning processes' which have their attendant pathologies.

Honneth's radicalisation of recognition was presented, however the continuing divergence in concerns between social pathology and recognition was underscored.

The second chapter offered a critique of the dominant Honnethian Critical Theory of Recognition by bringing Thompson's *The Domestication of Critical Theory* into dialogue with earlier critiques forwarded by McNay and Fraser. By engaging with critiques of recognition from across traditional disciplinary boundaries, I argued that the contemporary recognition paradigm has fundamental social-theoretical, political and philosophical weaknesses. Three central concerns of this analysis returned as motifs throughout the thesis: (a) the philosophical inadequacy of a neo-Idealist approach to the social world (from Thompson); (b) the dangers of championing a theoretical approach over and beyond its relevance to the context (from McNay), and, (c) a direct scepticism of any theorist who offers a form of critique which necessitates a 'monist' or unifocal perspective (from Fraser).

Chapter Three outlined how this restrictive recognition theoretical account has come to dominate social pathology scholarship. I argued that the framings of 'recognition' and 'social pathology' were fused by the Jyväskylä School's 'pathologies of recognition' approach to social theory and social research. I pointed to Honneth's framing of 'misdevelopments' as indicative of further attempts to restrict pathology diagnosing social critique, and to explicitly displace capital critique. Most importantly, I presented the increasingly prevalent 'recognition-cognitive' understanding of social pathology outlined by Zurn. I demonstrated how Zurn's framing, like the 'pathologies of recognition' approach, problematically excludes all non-recognition based understandings of social pathology. Further, I outlined how Zurn's radical cognitivism places further restrictions upon these already all-to-narrow parameters. It is only 'second-order disconnects' which should be understood *qua* social pathologies for Zurn. Such a framing is seen as restrictive even by those who otherwise advocate a recognition-theoretical model (Freyenhagen, 2015; Laitinen, 2015).

Having outlined the limitations of the dominant approach to engaging with social pathologies, the next three chapters sought to reconstruct efficacious framings of social pathology which have been displaced by the recognition-theoretical turn.

Chapter Four argued that a considered engagement with Rousseau discloses multiple, distinct framings of social pathology which transcend the recognition orthodoxy. It was particularly gratifying to discover such resources within Rousseau's work because Rousseau has been presented as the recognition theorist *par excellence* (Neuhouser, 2008). In Rousseau's analysis it is the foundational breach of the monological self-relation that led to the tragic loss of humankind's natural innocence. Yet, even for Rousseau, 'the father of recognition', a recognition optic, unaccompanied by alternate pathology framings, is of limited utility. I was thus pleased to locate numerous framings of social pathology that are anathema to a recognition perspective throughout Rousseau's work.

My fifth chapter presented the pathologies of reason approach. I argued that despite the philosophical complexity and the contested nature of the pathologies of reason perspective, there remains a real utility to this framework which is excluded by the recognition turn. This chapter reconstructed five different approaches to diagnosing pathologies of reason, seeking to draw out the shared understanding of reason in operation. Despite diverging philosophical convictions, all approaches presented shared a central dynamic and hold to an understanding of reason as 'thick' and 'social'. The chapter concluded by underscoring the utility of the pathologies of reason perspective, while furthering the argument that the restrictive 'recognition-cognitive' paradigm needs to be displaced.

Chapter Six presented the social theoretical infrastructure, and the substantive content, of Erich Fromm's diagnosis of 'pathological normalcy'. The chapter provided a sympathetic reconstruction of Fromm's framework, arguing that, when properly grasped, Fromm offers a valuable, consistent, and much needed, psychoanalytic-sociological dimension to discussions on social pathology. Having demonstrated the coherence and utility of Fromm's approach, this chapter once again served to demonstrate its exclusion from the dominant restrictive recognition-derived orthodoxy.

My seventh chapter argued that a reconfigured engagement with recognition could form part of a broader pathology diagnosing infrastructure. The chapter started by retracing the limitations of the dominant recognition paradigm which must be overcome for recognition insights to form part of a more inclusive Critical Theory. I then presented the utility harboured by the recognition approach that could potentially be extracted. In contrast to the dominant recognition framework which focuses on pathologically denied recognition, I argued that the true utility of the recognition approach lies as a means of engaging with pathological demands *for* recognition. From this perspective, a recognition approach is useful in that it presents a means of engaging with ideologically interpellated actors, whose claims for recognition reflect broader, pathological power relations dominant in the social order. The chapter thus argued that a cautious engagement with the recognition order has utility in that it can reflect the subject's petrification within ideology, and, therefore, offers an important entry point for engaging with the pathologies of the social world as part of a broader Critical Theoretical project.

Through the analysis developed across these seven chapters this thesis has argued that the dominant approach to engaging with social pathologies is problematically restrictive and philosophically unjustifiable. There are clearly many alternate framings of social pathology which offer utility to the Critical Theorist which are displaced by the exclusively recognition-derived approach to social pathology. This thesis thus functions as an intervention, seeking to challenge the dominant approach to social pathology scholarship, and, through doing so, seeks to contribute to the project of fighting back against the domestication of Critical Theory.

Conclusion

Critical Theory has lost perspective. It has retreated from the critique of capital and is increasingly mired in abstracted analytic philosophy, liberal-democratic theory, and neo-Idealism. In contrast, with a broader pathology diagnosing framework, Critical Theorists might once again have the tools to engage with the project's formative concerns: the critique of instrumental rationality, domination, and the ideological artifice which obscures comprehension of extractive and irrational dynamics. I submit that a polycentric pathology diagnosing framework, as advocated for in this thesis, can offer the foundations for timely social theoretical and social research contributions to this endeavour. The ability to diagnose social pathologies is an essential precondition for Critical Theorists being able to conceptualise and to challenge pressing manifest social irrationalities. The dominant recognition-derived framework is impotent, an obstacle to potent Critical Theoretical analysis. A turn to a broader engagement with pathology diagnosing social theory offers a means of combatting these developments. This thesis is thus submitted as one contribution among many to the project of transcending the domesticated state of contemporary Critical Theory.

References

Adorno T W (1978 [1951]) *Minima Moralia: Reflections from Damaged Life*. Translated by Jephcott E. London: Verso.

———. (1981 [1966] *Negative Dialectics*. Translated by Ashton E. London: Continuum.

Adorno T W, Adorno G, and Tiedeman R (1997 [1970]) *Aesthetic Theory*. Translated by Hullot-Kentor R. London: Athlone Press.

Adorno T W and Horkheimer M (1997 [1944]) *Dialectic of Enlightenment*. Translated by Cumming J. London: Verso.

Adorno T W et al (1994 [1950]) *The Authoritarian Personality*. New York City, NY: W W Norton and Company.

Affeldt S (1999) The Force of Freedom: Rousseau on Forcing to be Free. *Political Theory*. 27(99): 299-333.

Alanen L and Witt C (Eds.) (2004) *Feminist Reflections on the History of Philosophy*. Boston, MA: Kluwer Academic Publishers.

Alexander J C and Lara M P (1996) Honneth's new Critical Theory of Recognition. *New Left Review*. I (220): 126-136.

Allen A (2016) *The End of Progress: Decolonizing the Normative Foundations of Critical Theory*. New York City, NY: Columbia University Press.

Anderson J (1995 [1992]) Translator's Introduction. In Honneth A *The Struggle for Recognition*. Cambridge: Polity Press.

Antonovsky A (1996) The Salutogenic model as a theory to guide health promotion. *Health Promotion International*. 11(1): 11-18.

Aristotle (2009 [350BCE]) *Politics*. Translated by Stalley R and Barker E. Oxford: Oxford University Press.

Beck U (1997) Politics of Risk Society. In: Franklin J (Ed.) *The Politics of Risk Society*. Hoboken, NJ: Wiley, pp. 9-22.

Bell D (2018) The PowerPoint Philosophe: Waiting for Steven Pinker's Enlightenment. *The Nation*. Available online at: https://www.thenation.com/article/waiting-for-steven-pinkers-enlightenment/ [Accessed 7th October 2018].

Berlant L (2000) The Subject of True Feeling. In Ahmed S, Kilby J, Lury C, McNeil N and Skeggs B (Eds.) *Transformations: Thinking Through Feminism*. London: Routledge, pp. 32-47.

Berry D (2014) *Critical Theory and the Digital*. London: Bloomsbury.

Blackall E A (1959) *The Emergence of German as a Literary Language*. Cambridge: Cambridge University Press.

Bollenbeck G (forthcoming) Eine anerkennende Haltung annehmen! Verdinglichung „light". Über: Axel Honneth: Verdinglichung. *Sozialwissenschaftliche Literatur Rundschau*. 31(56). *Pagination forthcoming*.

Bonefeld W (2014) *Critical Theory and the Critique of Political Economy*. London: Bloomsbury.

Bookchin M (1962) *Our Synthetic Environment*. New York City: Knopf.

Borchers S (2006) *Hegel's Logic and Global Climate Change*. PhD Thesis. Nashville, TN: Vanderbilt University. (Subsequently published as *Hegel's Science of Logic and Global Climate Change: A Philosophical Explanation of an Environmental Crisis*. New York City, NY: Mellen Press.)

Bourdieu P (2000) *Pascalian Meditations*. Translated by Rafalko R. Cambridge: Polity Press.

Bowie A (2013) *Adorno and the Ends of Philosophy*. Cambridge: Polity Press.

Boyd R (2013) Economic Growth: A Social Pathology. *Resilience*. Available online at: https://www.resilience.org/stories/2013-11-08/economic-growth-a-social-pathology/ [Accessed 4th April 2019].

Bristow W F (2014) The Scandal of Hegel's Political Philosophy. In: Altman M C (Ed.) *The Palgrave Handbook of German Idealism*. London: Palgrave Macmillan, pp. 704-720.

Bronner S (2002) *Of Critical Theory and its Theorists*. Abingdon: Routledge.

———. (2011) *Critical Theory: A Very Short Introduction*. Oxford: Oxford University Press.

Brownestone S (2014) Whoops: Air Conditioning Is Making Cities Hotter, Not Colder. *Fast Company*. Published 6th November 2014. Available online at: https://www.fastcompany.com /3031696/whoops-air-conditioning-is-making-cities-hotter-not-colder. [Accessed 1st May 2019].

Buchwalter A (2016) The Concept of Normative Reconstruction: Honneth, Hegel, and the aims of a Critical Social Theory. In: Dahms H and Lybeck E (Eds.) *Reconstructing Social Theory, History and Practice*. Bingley, Yorks.: Emerald, pp. 57-88.

Buck-Morss S (2009) *Hegel, Haiti and Universal History*. Pittsburgh, PA: University of Pittsburgh Press.

Burnett J (2017) Racial Violence and the Brexit State. *Race and Class*. 58(4): 85-97.

Burston D (1991) *The Legacy of Erich Fromm*. Cambridge, MA: Harvard University Press.

Burston D and Olfman S (1996) Freud, Fromm and the Pathology of Normalcy. In: Cortina M and Maccoby M (Eds.) *A Prophetic Analyst: Erich Fromm's Contribution to Psychoanalysis*. Northvale, NJ: Jason Aronson, pp. 301-324.

Butler J (1997) *The Psychic Life of Power: Theories in Subjection*. Standford, CA: Standford University Press.

Butler J, Laclau E and Zizek S (2000) *Contingency, Hegemony, Universality: Contemporary Dialogues on the Left*. London: Verso.

Cajot J (1766) *Les Plagiats M. J. J. R. de Genève sur l'education*. Paris: Durand.

Caygill H (2004) Walter Benjamin's Concept of Cultural History. In Ferris D (Eds.) *The Cambridge Companion to Walter Benjamin*. Cambridge: Cambridge University Press, pp. 73-96.

Campbell S H (2012) *Rousseau and the Paradox of Alienation*. New York City, NY: Lexington Books.

Canivez P (2011) Pathologies of Recognition. *Philosophy and Social Criticism*. 37(8): 851-887.

———. (2019) The dialectic of recognition: A post-Hegelian approach. *European Journal of Social Theory*. 22(1): 63-79.

Celikates R (2018) *Critique as Social Practice: Critical Theory and Social Self-Understanding*. Translated by Van Steenberg N. New York City, NY: Rowman and Littlefield.

Chernilo D (2017) The question of the human in the Anthropocene debate. *European Journal of Social Theory*. 20(1): 44-60.

Chibber V (2013) *Postcolonial Theory and the Spectre of Capital*. London: Verso.

Chitty A (2018) Human Solidarity in Hegel and Marx. In Kandiyali J (Eds.) *Reassessing Marx's Social and Political Philosophy*. Abingdon: Routledge, pp. 128-154.

Code L (2008) Feminist Epistemologies and Women's Lives. In Alcoff L and Potter E (Eds.) *The Blackwell Guide to Feminist Philosophy*. New York City, NY: Wiley Blackwell, pp. 15-48.

Cohn D (2001) Does Socrates Speak for Plato? Reflections on an Open Question. *New Literary History*. 32(3): 485-500.

Connell R W (1987) *Gender and Power: Society, the Person, and Sexual Politics*. Cambridge: Polity Press.

Coulthard G (2014) *Red Skin, White Masks: Rejecting the Colonial Politics of Recognition*. Minneaopolis, MN: Minnesota University Press.

Cranston M (1997) *The Solitary Self: Jean-Jacques Rousseau in Exile and Adversity*. London: Penguin.

Cullen D (1993) *Freedom in Rousseau's Political Philosophy*. De Kalb, IL: Northern Illinois University Press.

Dagger R (1981) Understanding the General Will. *Western Political Science Quarterly*. 34(810): 359-371.

Dahbour O (2017) Totality, Reason, Dialectics: The Importance of Hegel for Critical Theory from Lukács to Honneth. In Thompson (Ed.) *The Palgrave Handbook of Critical Theory*. New York City, NY: Palgrave Macmillan, pp. 87-108.

Daly H (1996) *Beyond Growth*. Boston, MA: Beacon Press.

Damrosch L (2005) *Jean-Jacques Rousseau: Restless Genius*. Boston, MA: Mariner Books.

Darling J (1994) *Child Centred Education and its Critics*. London: Paul Chapman Publishing.

Darwin C (2004 [1871]) *The Descent of Man: Selection in Relation to Sex*. London: Penguin.

Dawson A (2019) *Extreme Cities: The Peril and Promise of Urban Life in the Age of Climate Change*. London: Verso.

de Boer K (2013) Beyond Recognition? Critical Reflections on Honneth's Reading of Hegel's Philosophy of Right. *International Journal of Philosophical Studies*. 21(4): 534-558.

Delaney J (2009) *Starting with Rousseau.* London: Continuum.

Della Volpe G (1979) *Rousseau and Marx*. Translated by Fraser J. Atlantic Highlands, N.J.: Humanities Press.

Delanty G (2009) *The Cosmopolitan Imagination: The Renewal of Critical Social Theory.* Cambridge: Cambridge University Press.

———. (2011) Varieties of critique in sociological theory and their methodological implications for social research. *Irish Journal of Sociology.* 19(1): 68-92.

Delanty G and Harris N (2018) The idea of Critical Cosmopolitanism. In: Delanty G (Ed.) *The Routledge Handbook of Cosmopolitan Studies.* Abingdon: Routledge, pp. 113-122.

Deranty J-P (2009) *Beyond Communication: A Critical Study of Axel Honneth's Social Philosophy.* Leiden: Brill.

Deutscher P and Lafont C (Eds.) (2017) *Critical Theory in Critical Times: Transforming the Global Political and Economic Order*. New York City, NY: Columbia University Press.

Douglass R (2015) *Rousseau and Hobbes: Nature, Free Will, and the Passions*. Oxford: Oxford University Press.

Dreyfus H and Rabinow P (1982) *Michel Foucault: Beyond Structuralism and Hermeneutics.* Brighton: Harvester.

Du Bois W E B (2016) *The Souls of Black Folk*. London: Dover Thrift.

Durant W and Durant A (1967) *The Story of Civilization: Rousseau and Revolution; a history of civilization in France, England, and Germany from 1756, and in the remainder of Europe from 1715 to 1789.* New York: Simon and Schuster.

Durkheim E (1960) *Montesquieu and Rousseau: Forerunners of sociology*. Translated by Manheim R. Ann Arbor, MI: University of Michigan Press.

Durkin K (2014) *The Radical Humanism of Erich Fromm*. New York City, NY: Palgrave Macmillan.

———. (2019) Erich Fromm and Theodor W. Adorno Reconsidered: A Case Study in Intellectual History. *New German Critique*. 46(1): 103-126.

Eder K (1985) *Geschichte als Lernprozess? Zur Pathogenese politischer Modernität in Deutschland*. Frankfurt am Main: Suhrkamp.

Elmgren H (2015) Recognition and the Ideology of Merit. *Studies in Social and Political Thought*. 25(1): 152-173.

Fanon F (1952) *Black Skin, White Masks*. Translated by Markmann C. London: Pluto.

Ferrara A (2017) *Rousseau and Critical Theory*. Leiden: Brill.

Feuerbach L (2008 [1841]) *The Essence of Christianity*. Translated by Eliot G. New York City, NY: Dover Publications.

Foucault M (1975) *Discipline and Punish*. Translated by Sheridan A. London: Penguin.

———. (2003 [1963]) *The Birth of the Clinic: An Archaeology of Medical Perception*. Translated by Sheridan A. London: Routledge.

Fraser N (1995a) From redistribution to recognition? Dilemmas of Justice in a 'Post-Socialist' Age. *New Left Review* I/212: 68-93.

———. (1995b) 'Recognition or redistribution? A critical reading of Iris Young's *Justice and the Politics of Difference*'. *The Journal of Political Philosophy*. 3(2): 166-180.

———. (1997) A Rejoinder to Iris Marion Young. *New Left Review*, I/223: 126-129.

Fraser N and Honneth A (2001) *Redistribution or Recognition? A Political-Philosophical Exchange*. Translated by Golb J, Ingram J and Wilke C. London: Verso.

Fraser N and Jaeggi R (2018) *Capitalism: A Conversation in Critical Theory*. Cambridge and Medford, MA: Polity.

Frega R (2014) Between Pragmatism and Critical Theory: Social Philosophy Today. *Human Studies*. 37(1): 57-82.

Freud S (1953) *Civilisation and Its Discontents*. Translated by Riviere J. London: Hogarth Press.

———. (1959) *Civilized Sexual Morality and Modern Nervous Illness*. Translated by Strachey J, Freud A, Strachey A and Tyson A. London: Read Books.

Freundlieb D (2015) Why Subjectivity Matters: Critical Theory and the Philosophy of the Subject. *Critical Horizons*. 1(2): 229-245.

Freyenhagen F (2013) *Adorno's Practical Philosophy: Living Less Wrongly*. Cambridge: Cambridge University Press.

———. (2015) Honneth on Social Pathologies: A Critique. *Critical Horizons* 16(2): 131-152.

Fromm E (1941) *Escape From Freedom*. New York: Farrar and Rinehart.

———. (1944) Individual and social origins of neurosis. *American Sociology Review*. IX(4): 380-384.

———. (1963 [1955]) *The Sane Society*. Translated by Rotten E. New York: Rinehart and Winston.

———. (1979) *To Have or to Be?* London: Abacus.

———. (1983 [1962]) *Beyond The Chains of Illusion: My Encounter with Marx & Freud*. London: Abacus.

———. (2010 [1991]) *The Pathology of Normalcy*. Riverdale, NY: AMHF.

Fuchs C (2018) *Digital Demagogue: Capitalism in the Age of Trump and Twitter*. London: Pluto Press.

Funk R (2000 [1999]) *Erich Fromm: His Life and Ideas*. New York: Continuum.

———. (2010 [1991]) 'Introduction' in Fromm E *The Pathology of Normalcy*. Riverdale, NY: AMHF.

Gallie W (1956) Essentially Contested Concepts. *Proceedings of the Aristotelian Society*. 56: 97-114.

Gay P (1959) *Voltaire's Politics: The Poet as Realist*. New Jersey: Princeton University Press.

Gibbon E (1996) *The History of the Decline and Fall of the Roman Empire: Vol. 1*. London: Penguin.

Gleeson L (2015) Review of Freedom's Right by Axel Honneth. *Studies in Social and Political Thought*, 25(1): 254-259.

Gray J (2018) Unenlightened thinking: Steven Pinker's embarrassing new book is a feeble sermon for rattled liberals. *New Statesman*. Published online 22nd February 2018. Available online at: https://www.newstatesman.com/culture/books/2018/02/unenlightened-thinking-steven-pinker-s-embarrassing-new-book-feeble-sermon [Accessed 7th October 2018].

Grierson J (2018) Hostile environment: anatomy of a policy disaster. *The Guardian*. 27th August 2018. Available online at: https://www.theguardian.com/uk-news/2018/aug/27/hostile-environment-anatomy-of-a-policy-disaster [Accessed 14th April 2019].

Groddeck G (1929) *The Unknown Self: A New Psychological Approach to the Problems of Life, with Special Reference to Disease*. Translated by Collins V M E. London: The C.W. Daniel Company.

———. (1977) *The Meaning of Illness*. Translated by Schacht L. Madison, CT: International Universities Press.

———. (2012 [1913]) *Der gesunde und kranke Mensch*. Mannheim: Outlook Verlag.

———. (2013 [1933]) *Exploring the Unconscious: Further Exercises in Applied Analytical Psychology*. Eastford, CT: Martino Fine Books.

Grollios V (2017) *Negativity and Democracy: Marxism and the Critical Theory Tradition*. Abingdon: Routledge.

Guess R (2004) Dialectics and the Revolutionary Impulse. In: Rush F (Ed.) (2004) *The Cambridge Companion to Critical Theory*. Cambridge: Cambridge University Press, pp. 103-138.

Habermas J (1982) The Entwinement of Myth and Enlightenment: Rereading dialectic of Enlightenment. Translated by Levin T. *New German Critique*. 26(1): 13-30.

———. (1984) *The Theory of Communicative Action*. Translated by McCarthy T. Boston, MA: Beacon Press.

———. (1987 [1968]) *Knowledge and Human Interests*. Translated by Shapiro J. Cambridge: Polity.

———. (2000 [1992]) *Postmetaphysical Thinking: Philosophical Essays*. Translated by Hohengarten W M. Cambridge, MA: MIT Press.

———. (2001) *On the Pragmatics of Social Interaction: Preliminary Studies in the Theory of Communicative Action*. Translated by Fultner B. Cambridge, MA: MIT Press.

———. (2017a) An Exploration of the Meaning of Transnationalization of Democracy, Using the Example of the European Union. In: Deutscher P and Lafont C (Eds.) *Critical Theory in Critical Times: Transforming the Global Political and Economic Order*. New York City, NY: Columbia University Press, pp. 3-18.

———. (2017b) *Postmetaphysical Thinking II*. Translated by Cronin C. Cambridge: Polity.

Hall J (1973) *Rousseau: An Introduction to His Political Philosophy*. Plymouth: The Bowering Press.

Han B (2012) *The Agony of Eros: Volume 1 (Untimely Meditations)*. Translated by Butler E. London: MIT Press.

Hardimon M O (1992) The Project of Reconciliation: Hegel's Social Philosophy. *Philosophy and Public Affairs*. 21(2): 165-195.

Harding S (2004) *The Feminist Standpoint Theory Reader: Intellectual and Political Controversies*. London: Routledge.

Harraway D (1988) Situated Knowledges: The Science Question in Feminism and the Privilege of Partial Perspective. *Feminist Studies*. 14(3): 575-599.

Harris H S (1958) Hegelianism of the 'Right' and 'Left'. *The Review of Metaphysics*. 11(4): 603-609.

Harris N (2018a) Book Review: Critical Theory in Critical Times: Transforming the Global Political and Economic Order. *European Journal of Social Theory*. 21(4): 569-573.

———. (2018b) Book Review: Critique as Social Practice: Critical Theory and Social Self Understanding. *European Journal of Social Theory*. 22(1): 123-126.

———. (2019) Pathologies of Recognition: An Introduction. *European Journal of Social Theory*. 22(1): 3-9.

Harvey D (2017) *Marx, Capital and the Madness of Economic Reason*. London: Profile Books.

Haym R (1857) *Hegel Und Seine Zeit*. Hildesheim: Georg Olms Verlagsbuchhandlung.

Hegel G W F (1953 [1822]) *Reason in History: General Introduction to the Philosophy of History.* Translated by Hartman R. Indianapolis, IN: Bobbs-Merrill.

———. (1970 [1807]) *Phenomenology of Spirit.* Translated by Miller A V. Oxford: Oxford University Press.

———. (1979 [1802]) *System of Ethical Life.* Translated by Knox T. Albany: State University of New York Press.

———. (1991 [1820]) *Philosophy of Right.* Translated by Nesbit H B. Cambridge: Cambridge University Press.

———. (2015 [1816]) *Science of Logic.* Translated by Di Giovanni G. Cambridge: Cambridge University Press.

Held D (2013) *Introduction to Critical Theory: Horkheimer to Habermas.* Hoboken, NY: Wiley.

Herf J (2012) Dialectic of Enlightenment Reconsidered. *New German Critique.* 39(3): 81-89.

Heywood A (2007) *Political Ideologies: An Introduction.* Basingstoke: Palgrave MacMillan.

Hirvonen O (2015) Pathologies of Collective Recognition. *Studies in Social and Political Thought.* 25(1): 209-226.

Hirvonen O and Pennanen J (2019) Populism as a Pathological form of Politics of Recognition. *European Journal of Social Theory.* 22(1): 27-44.

Holloway J Matamoros F and Tischler S (2009) *Negativity and Revolution: Adorno and Political Activism.* London: Pluto Press.

Honneth A (1991 [1985]) *The Critique of Power: Reflective Stages in a Critical Social Theory.* Translated by Baynes K. Cambridge: MIT Press.

———. (1995 [1992]) *The Struggle for Recognition.* Translated by Anderson J. Cambridge: Polity Press.

———. (2000) The Possibility of a Disclosing Critique of Society: The Dialectic of Enlightenment in Light of Current Debates in Social Criticism. *Constellations* 7(1): 116-127.

———. (2003) 'Anxiety and Politics': The Strengths and Weaknesses of Franz Neumann's Diagnosis of a Social Pathology. *Constellations* 10(2): 247-255.

———. (2004a) A Social Pathology of Reason: On the Intellectual Legacy of Critical Theory. In: Rush F (ed.) *The Cambridge Companion to Critical Theory*. Cambridge: Cambridge University Press, pp. 19-42.

———. (2004b) Organized Self-Realization: some paradoxes of Individualization. *European Journal of Social Theory*. 7(4): 463-478.

———. (2007a) *Disrespect: The Normative Foundations of Critical Theory*. Cambridge: Polity Press.

———. (2007b) *Pathologies of Reason: On the Legacy of Critical Theory*. Translated by Ingram J. New York City, NY: Columbia University Press.

———. (2007c) Pathologies of the Social: The Past and Present of Social Philosophy. In: *Disrespect: The Normative Foundations of Critical Theory*. Translated by Ganahal J. Cambridge: Polity Press, pp. 3-49.

———. (2007d) The irreducibility of Progress: Kant's Account of the Relationship between Morality and History. *Critical Horizons*. 8(1): 1-17.

———. (2008) *Reification: A New Look at an Old Idea*. Oxford: Oxford University Press.

———. (2010) *The Pathologies of Individual Freedom*. Translated by Löb L. Princeton, NJ: Princeton University Press.

———. (2014a) The Diseases of Society: Approaching a Nearly Impossible Concept. Translated by Särkelä A. *Social Research*. 81(3): 683-703.

———. (2014b [2011]) *Freedom's Right*. Translated by Ganahal J. Cambridge: Polity Press.

———. (2016) *The Idea of Socialism: Towards a Renewal*. Translated by Ganahl J. Cambridge: Polity Press.

Horkheimer M (1975 [1937]) Tradition and Critical Theory. In: *Critical Theory: Selected Essays*. Translated by Herder and Herder. New York City, NY: Continuum, pp. 188-244.

———. (1993) Reason Against Itself: Some Remarks on Enlightenment. *Theory, Culture and Society*. (10): 79-88.

———. (2014 [1967]) *Critique of Instrumental Reason*. Translated by O'Connell M. London: Continuum.

Houlgate S (2012) *Hegel's Phenomenology of Spirit: A Reader's Guide*. London: Bloomsbury.

Howitt W (1840) *Visits to Remarkable Places: old halls, battle fields and scenes illustrative of striking passages in English History and Poetry*. London: Longman, Orme, Brown, Green and Longmans.

Hoy D C and McCarthy T (1994) *Critical Theory*. Oxford: Blackwell.

Hulliung M (1994) *The Autocritique of Enlightenment: Rousseau and the Philosophes*. Cambridge, MA: Harvard University Press.

Ikäheimo H (2007) Recognizing Persons. *Journal of Consciousness Studies*. 14(5-6): 224-247.

———. (2002) On the Genesis and Species of Recognition. *Inquiry*. 45: 447-462.

Ingleby D (2002 [1991]) Introduction to the Second Edition. In: Fromm S *The Sane Society*. Abingdon, Oxon: Routledge, pp. xv-liv.

Ingram D (2010) Recognition Within the Limits of Reason: Remarks on Pippin's Hegel's Practical Philosophy. *Inquiry* (5): 470-489.

Jaeggi R (2016) *Alienation*. Translated by Neuhouser F. New York City, NY: Columbia University Press.

———. (2018) *On the Critique of Forms of Life*. Translated by Cronin C. Cambridge, MA: Harvard University Press.

James D (2013) *Rousseau and German Idealism: Freedom, Dependence and Necessity*. Cambridge: Cambridge University Press.

Jay M. (1996 [1973]) *The Dialectical Imagination: A History of the Frankfurt School and Institute of Social Research, 1923-1950*. Berkeley, CA: University of California Press.

———. (2008) Introduction. In: Honneth A *Reification: A New Look at an Old Idea*. Oxford: Oxford University Press, pp. 3-16.

———. (2016) *Reason After Its Eclipse: On Late Critical Theory*. Milwaukee, WI: University of Wisconsin University Press.

Jeffries S (2017) *Grand Hotel Abyss: The Lives of the Frankfurt School*. London: Verso.

Jütten T (2017) Dignity, Esteem, and Social Contribution: A Recognition-Theoretical View. *Journal of Political Philosophy.* 25(3): 259-280.

Kant I (1996 [1798]) An answer to the question: what is Enlightenment? in Gregor M (Eds.) (1996) *Immanuel Kant. Practical Philosophy.* Translated by Gregor M. Cambridge: Cambridge University Press.

Kapoor N (2013) The advancement of racial neoliberalism in Britain. *Ethnic and Racial Studies.* 36(6): 1028-1046.

Kelly G (1966) Notes on Hegel's 'Lordship and Bondage'. *The Review of Metaphysics.* 19(4): 780-802.

Klein N (2014) *This Changes Everything: Capitalism vs. The Climate.* New York: Simon and Schuster.

Kok A and van Houdt J (2014) *Reconsidering the Origins of Recognition: New Perspectives on German Idealism.* Newcastle-upon-Tyne: Cambridge Scholars.

Krishnamurti J (2008 [1962]) *Krishnamurti's Notebook.* Ojal, CA: K Publications.

Kubrick S (1964) *Dr. Strangelove or: How I learned to Stop Worrying and Love the Bomb* [Film]. Los Angeles, CA: Columbia Pictures.

Kunstler J (2012) *Too Much Magic: Wishful Thinking, Technology, and the Fate of the Nation.* New York, NY: Atlantic Monthly Press.

Lacan J (1975) *Le Seminaire Livre XX, Encore (1972-3).* Translated by Miller J. Paris: Seuil.

Laegaard S (2005) On the prospects for a liberal theory of recognition. *Res Publica.* 11: 325-348.

Laitinen A (2015) Social Pathologies, Reflexive Pathologies, and the Idea of Higher-Order Disorders. *Studies in Social and Political* Thought, 25(1): 44-65.

Laitinen A and Ikäheimo H (2011) *Recognition and Social Ontology.* Leiden: Brill.

Laitinen A and Särkelä A (2019) Four Conceptions of Social Pathology. *European Journal of Social Theory.* 22(1): 80-102.

Laitinen A, Särkelä A and Ikäheimo H (2015) Pathologies of Recognition: An Introduction. *Studies in Social and Political Thought.* 25(1): 1-24.

Lear E (1870) *Journal of a Landscape Painter in Corsica*. London: Robert John Bush.

Lenin V I (1972) *Collected Works.* Translated by Dutt C. Moscow: Progress Publishers.

———. (1977) *Collected Works.* Translated by Hanna G. Moscow: Progress Publishers.

Lukacs G (1972 [1923]) *History and Class Consciousness: Studies in Marxist Dialectics.* Translated by Livingstone R. Cambridge, MA: The MIT Press.

Lyotard J F (1984 [1979]) *The Postmodern Condition: A Report on Knowledge*. Translated by Bennington G and Massumi B. Manchester: Manchester University Press.

MacLay G R (1990) *The Social Organism: A Short History of the Idea that a Human Society May be Regarded as a Gigantic Living Creature*. Great Barrington, MA.: North River Press.

Malm A (2016) *Fossil Capital: The Rise of Steam Power and the Roots of Global Warming*. London: Verso.

Marcuse F (1969 [1941]) *Reason and Revolution: Hegel and the Rise of Social Theory*. London: Routledge and Kegan Paul.

———. (1964) *One Dimensional Man*. Boston, MA: Beacon Press.

Margolies R (1996) Self Development and Psychotherapy in a Period of Rapid Social Change. In: Cortina M and Maccoby M (Eds.) *A Prophetic Analyst: Erich Fromm's contribution to psychoanalysis*. Northvale, NJ: Jason Aronson, pp 361-401.

Martineau W, Meer N and Thompson S (2012) Theory and Practice in the Politics of Recognition and Misrecognition. *Res Publica*. 18(1): 1-9.

Marx K and Engels F (1939 [1932]) *German Ideology*. Translated by Pascal R. New York City, NY: International Publishers.

Marx K (1844) Letter from Marx to Ruge. First published in *Deutsch-Französische Jahrbücher*. Available online at Marxists.org at https://www.marxists.org/archive/marx/works/1843/letters/43_ 09-alt. htm [Accessed 13th January 2019].

———. (1959 [1843-4]) Toward the Critique of Hegel's Philosophy of Right. Translated by Feuer L. In: Feuer L (Ed.) *Marx and Engels: Basic Writings on Politics and Philosophy.* New York City, NY: Doubleday Anchor Original.

———. (1959 [1844]) *Economic and Philosophical Manuscripts of 1844*. Translated by Milligan M. Moscow: Progress.

———. (1973 [1939]) *Grundrisse*: *Foundations of the critique of political economy*. Translated by Nicolaus M. New York City, NY: Vintage Books.

———. (1976 [1867]) *Capital Volume 1*. Translated by Fowkes B. London: Penguin.

———. (2010) A Contribution to the Critique of Political Economy. In: Sitton J F. (Eds.) Marx Today. New York City, NY: Palgrave MacMillan, pp. 91-94.

McGee V (1991) *Truth, Vagueness, and Paradox: An Essay on the Logic of Truth*, Indianapolis, IN: Hackett Publishing.

McLellan D (1985 [1973]) *Karl Marx: His Life and Thought*. London and Basingstoke: MacMillan.

McNay L (2008) *Against Recognition*. Cambridge: Polity Press.

Mecklin J (Eds.) (2008) It is 2 minutes to midnight. *Bulletin of the Atomic Scientists*. Available online at: https://thebulletin.org/sites/default/files/2018%20Doomsday%20Clock%20 Statement.pdf [Accessed 13th March 2019].

Mehrotra S (1991) On the Social Specifications of Use Value in Marx's Capital. *Social Scientist*. 19(8/9): 72-77.

Melzer A (2006) The Origin of the counter-Enlightenment: Rousseau and the new religion of sincerity. In: Scott J (Ed.) *Jean-Jacques Rousseau: Critical Assessments of Leading Political Philosophers*. London: Routledge.

Miller J (1974) *Psychoanalysis and Women*. London: Pelican,

———. (1984) *Rousseau: Dreamer of Democracy*. New Haven, CT: Yale University Press.

Mittlemark M B (2016) Introduction to the Handbook of Salutogenesis. In: Mittelmark M B, Sagy S, Eriksson M, Bauer G, Pelikan J, Lindstrom B and Espnes G (Eds.) *The Handbook of Salutogenesis*. New York City, NY: Springer.

Monbiot G (2017) *How Did We Get Into This Mess?* London: Verso.

———. You can deny environmental calamity – until you check the facts. *The Guardian*. Published 7th March 2018. Available online at: https://www.theguardian.com/comm

entisfree/2018/mar/07/environmental-calamity-facts-steven-pinker   [Accessed   7th October 2018].

Myers R (2009) Philosophy and Rhetoric in Rousseau's "First Discourse". *Philosophy and Rhetoric.* 28(3): 199-214.

Naess A (1989) *Ecology, Community and Lifestyle.* Cambridge: Cambridge University Press.

———. (2008) *Ecology of Wisdom.* London: Penguin.

Nájera R (2017) Scholastic Philosophers on the Role of the Body in Knowledge. In: Smith J (Eds.) *Embodiment: A History.* Oxford: Oxford University Press.

Neuhouser F (1993) Freedom, Dependence and the General Will. *The Philosophical Review.* 102(3): 363-395.

———. (2008) *Rousseau's Theodicy of Self-Love: Evil, Rationality, and the Drive for Recognition.* Oxford: Oxford University Press.

———. (2012) Rousseau und die Idee einer pathologischen Gesellschaft. Translated by Neuhouser F. *Politische Vierteljahresschrift* 53(4): 628-745.

———. (2018) Nietzsche on Spiritual Health and Cultural Pathology. In: Katsafanas P (Ed.) (2018) *The Nietzschean Mind.* London: Routledge, pp. 334-347.

Niemi P (2015) The Professional Form of Recognition in Social Work. *Studies in Social and Political Thought.* 25(1): 174-190.

Noone J B (1980) *Rousseau's Social Contract.* Athens, GA: University of Georgia Press.

Novack G and Mandel E (1973) *The Marxist Theory of Alienation.* Vancouver, BC: Pathfinder.

O'Connor B (2004) *Adorno's Negative Dialectic: Philosophy and the Possibility of Critical Rationality.* London: MIT Press.

O'Hara L and Gregg J (2012) Human Rights Casualties from the "war on obesity": Why focusing on body weight is inconsistent with a human rights approach to health. *Fat Studies.* 1: 32-46.

O'Neill S and Smith N (Eds.) (2012) *Recognition Theory as Social Research.* Basingstoke: Palgrave Macmillan.

O'Sullivan L (2016) The Idea of a Category Mistake: From Ryle to Habermas, and Beyond. *History of European Ideas*. 42(2): 178-194.

Ollmann B (1971) *Alienation: Marx's Concept of Man in Capitalist Society*. Cambridge: Cambridge University Press.

Ollmann B (2003) *Dance of the Dialectic: Steps in Marx's Method*. Champaign, IL: University of Illinois Press.

Osborne P and Dews P (1987) The Frankfurt School and the Problem of Critique. A reply to McCartney. *Radical Philosophy*. 45(1): 2-11.

Petherbridge D (Eds.) (2011) *Axel Honneth: Critical Essays: with a reply by Axel Honneth*. Leiden: Brill.

Pierre-Louis K (2018) The World Wants Air-Conditioning. The Could Warm the World. *The New York Times*. Published 15th May 2018. Available online at: https://www.nytimes.com /2018/05/15/climate/air-conditioning.html [Accessed 1st May 2019].

Piketty T (2014) *Capital in the Twenty-First Century*. Translated by Goldhammer A. Cambridge, MA: The Belknap Press.

Pinker S (2003) *The Blank Slate: The Modern Denial of Human Nature*. London: Penguin.

———. (2018) *Enlightenment Now: The Case for Reason, Science, Humanism, and Progress*. London: Allen Lane.

Pippin R (1981) Hegel's Political Argument and the Problem of Verwirklichung. *Political Theory*. 9(4): 509-532.

Plato (1979 [c.399BCE]) *Apology of Socrates*. Translated by Thomas G. Ithaca, NY: Cornell University Press.

———. (2008 [380BCE]) *Republic*. Oxford: Oxford University Press.

Plattner M F (1979) *Rousseau's State of Nature: An Interpretation of the Discourse on Inequality*. DeKalb, IL: Northern Illinois University Press.

Pollock F (1941) State Capitalism: Its Possibilities and Limitations. *Studies in Political and Social Science*. 9(2): 200-225.

Popper K (1945) *The Open Society and its Enemies*. Abingdon: Routledge.

Ransby B (2015) The Class Politics of Black Lives Matter. *Dissent.* Available online at: https://www.dissentmagazine.org/article/class-politics-black-lives-matter [Accessed 28th February 2019].

Ratner C (2014) Pathological Normalcy: A Construct for Comprehending and Overcoming Psychological Aspects of Alienation. *The Humanistic Psychologist.* 42: 298-303.

———. (2019) *Neoliberal Psychology.* New York, NY: Springer.

Ricoeur P (2005) *The Course of Recognition.* Cambridge, MA: Harvard University Press.

Ritter A and Bondanella J C (Eds.) (1988) *Rousseau's Political Writings.* Translated by Bondanella J C. New York: W W Norton and Company.

Roberts J (2004) The Dialectic of Enlightenment. In: Rush F (Eds) (2004) *The Cambridge Companion to Critical Theory.* Cambridge: Cambridge University Press.

Robinson P (2008) Jean-Jacques Rousseau and history: moral truth at the expense of facticity. *Rethinking History.* 12(3): 417-431.

Rousseau J-J (1911 [1762]) *Émile, or On Education.* Translated by Foxley B. London: Everyman's Library.

———. (1950 [1752]) *Le Devin du Village.* New York: E F Calmus.

———. (1953 [1782]) *The Confessions.* Translated by Cohen J. London: Penguin.

———. (1960 [1758]) *Letter to d'Alembert.* Translated by Bloom A. Ithaca, NY: Cornell University Press.

———. (1968a [1762]) *The Social Contract.* Translated by Cranston M. London: Penguin.

———. (1968b [1782]) Considerations on the Government of Poland. In: Watkins F (Eds.) *Jean Jacques Rousseau Political Writings.* Translated by Watkins F. Madison, WI: University of Wisconsin Press, pp. 156-267.

———. (1978 [1758]) (Discourse on) Political Economy. Translated by Masters J. In: Masters R (Ed.) *On the Social Contract, with Geneva Manuscript and Political Economy.* New York City, NY: St. Martin's Press.

———. (1979 [1782]) *Reveries of the Solitary Walker.* Translated by France P. London: Penguin.

———. (1984 [1762]) *Discourse on the Origins of Inequality*. Translated by Cranston M. London: Penguin.

———. (1986 [1768]) Constitutional Project for Corsica. In: Watkins F (Eds.) *Jean Jacques Rousseau Political Writings*. Translated by Watkins F. Madison, WI: University of Wisconsin Press.

———. (1990 [1761]) The State of War. Translated by Roosevelt G. In: Roosevelt G (1990) *Reading Rousseau in the Nuclear Age*. Philadelphia, PA: Temple University Press.

———. (1993 [1750]) A Discourse on the Arts and Sciences. Translated by Cole G D H. In: Rousseau J-J (1993) *The Social Contract and Discourses*. London: Everyman, pp. 125-155.

———. (1995 [1753]) Letter on French Music. In: Gagnebin B, Raynard M et al (Eds.) (1995) *Rousseau's Oeuvres Completes*. Gallimond: Bibliotheque de la Pleide.

———. (1997a [1755]) Rousseau J-J (1997) *The Discourses and Other Early Writings*. Translated by Gourevitch V. Cambridge: Cambridge University Press.

———. (1997b [1761]) *Julie, or the New Heloise: Letters of Two Lovers Who Live in a Small Town at the Foot of the Alps*. Translated by Vaché J and Stewart P. Hanover and London: University Press of New England.

———. (1997c [1781]) Essays on the Origins of Language. In: Gourevitch V (Eds.) *Rousseau's Discourses and Other Early Writings*. Translated by Gourevitch V. Cambridge: Cambridge University Press, pp. 257-310.

Rousseliere G (2016) Rousseau on Freedom in Commercial Society. *American Journal of Political Science*. 60(2): 352-363.

Rush F (2013) Rationalisation, Reification, Instrumental Reason. In Walker J (Ed.) *The Impact of Idealism: The legacy of post-Kantian German thought*, Volume II: Historical, Social and Political Thought. Cambridge: Cambridge University Press, pp. 186-207.

Russell B (2015 [1946]) *A History of Western Philosophy*. London: Routledge.

Ryle G (2002 [1949]) *The Concept of Mind*. Chicago: University of Chicago Press.

Said E (1993) *Culture and Imperialism*. New York City, NY: Vintage Books.

———. (2003 [1978]) *Orientalism*. London: Penguin.

Santayana G (1916) *Egotism in German Philosophy*. London: J M Dent and Sons.

Schaub J (2015) Misdevelopments, pathologies, and normative revolutions: Normative Reconstruction as method of critical theory. *Critical Horizons*. 16(2): 107-130.

Schaub J and Odigbo M (2019) Expanding the Taxonomy of (Mis-)Recognition in the Economic Sphere. *European Journal of Social Theory*. 22(1): 103-122.

Schecter D (2010) *The Critique of Instrumental Reason from Weber to Habermas*. London: Continuum.

Schopenhaeur A (1909) *The World as Will and Representation*. Translated by Haldane R B and Kemp J. London: Kegan Paul.

Selby J (1993) Psychoanalysis as a Critical Theory of Gender. In: Stam H J, Mos P L, Thorngate W and Kaplan B (Eds). *Recent Trends in Theoretical Psychology*. New York City, NY: Springer, pp. 307-318.

Sewell D (2009) *The Political Gene: How Darwin's Ideas Changed Politics,* London: Palgrave MacMillan.

Shaver R (1989) Rousseau and Recognition. *Social Theory and Practice*. 15(3): 261-283.

Siddique H (2018) Tories have avoided the truth over austerity and food banks. *The Guardian*. 1st August 2018. Available online at: https://www.theguardian.com/society/2018/aug/01/tories-have-avoided-the-truth-over-austerity-and-food-banks [Accessed 4th April 2019].

Simmel G (2011 [1900]) *The Philosophy of Money*. London: Routledge.

Simon-Ingram J (1991) Alienation, Individuation, and Enlightenment in Rousseau's Social Theory. *Eighteenth-Century Studies*. 24(3): 315-335.

Sloterdijk P (2012) *The Art of Philosophy: Wisdom as a Practice*. New York, NY: Columbia University Press.

Solomon R C (1970) Hegel's Concept of 'Geist'. *The Review of Metaphysics*. 23(4) 642-661.

Sorenson L (1990) Natural Inequality and Rousseau's Political Philosophy in his Discourse on Inequality. *Political Research Quarterly* (90)43: 763-788.

Stan H and Montgomery L (2017) Reflecting Critically on Contemporary Social Pathologies: social work and the 'good life'. *Critical and Radical Social Work*. 5(2): 181-196.

Stern D (1977) *The First Relationship: Mother and Infant*. London: Open Books.

Stern R (2009) *Hegelian Metaphysics*. Oxford: Oxford University Press.

Stewart P and Vaché J (1997) Introduction. In Rousseau J-J (1997 [1761]) *Julie, or the New Heloise: Letters of Two Lovers Who Live in a Small Town at the Foot of the Alps*. Translated by Vaché J and Stewart P. London: University Press of New England, pp. i-xxxi.

Streeck W (2016) *How Will Capitalism End?* London: Verso.

Strong T B (1994) *Jean-Jacques Rousseau: The Politics of the Ordinary*. London: Sage.

Struve T (1978) *Die Entwicklung der organologischen Staatsauffas-sung im Mittelater*. Stuttgart: Hiersemann.

Strydom P (2008) 'Immanent Transcendence: Critical Theory's Left-Hegelian Heritage'. Conference Paper Presented for the European Journal of Social Theory's 10th Anniversary at the University of Sussex, 'Europe since 1989'. Presented 19-21st June 2008. Available online at: https://www.researchgate.net/publication/301229835_Immanent_Transcendence_Critical_Th eory's_Left-Hegelian_Heritage [Accessed 1st April 2019].

———. (2011) *Contemporary Critical Theory and Methodology*. Abingdon: Routledge.

———. (2017) Infinity, infinite processes and limit concepts: Recovering a Neglected background of social and critical theory. *Philosophy and Social Criticism*. 43(8): 793-811.

———. (2018) Inferential Dialectics: On Dialectical Reasoning in Critical Social Science and the Sociocultural World. In: Giri A (Ed.) *Beyond Sociology: Trans-Civilizational Dialogues and Planetary Conversations*. Singapore: Palgrave MacMillan, pp. 71-92.

Stuckler D (2013) *The Body Economic: Why Austerity Kills*, New York City, NY: Basic Books.

Taylor C (1994) The Politics of Recognition. In: Gutmann A (Ed.) *Multiculturalism: Examining the Politics of Recognition*. Princeton, NJ: Princeton University Press, pp. 25-73.

Thompson A (2009) *Erich Fromm: Shaper of the Human Condition*. Basingstoke: Palgrave Macmillan.

Thompson M J (2014) Normative Humanism as Redemptive Critique. In: Miri S J, Lake R and Kress T M (Eds.) *Reclaiming the Sane Society*. Boston, MA: Sense, pp. 37-58.

———. (2015) *Rousseau and the Origins of Critical Theory*. Paper delivered at the International Social Theory Consortium, King's College, Cambridge. 17th June 2015.

———. (2016) *The Domestication of Critical Theory.* London: Rowman and Littlefield.

———. (2017) The Failure of the Recognition Paradigm in Critical Theory. In: Schmitz V (Ed.) *Axel Honneth and the Critical Theory of Recognition.* Basingstoke: Palgrave Macmillan, pp. 243-272.

———. (2019) Hierarchy, Social Pathology and the Failure of Recognition Theory. *European Journal of Social Theory.* 22(1): 10-26.

Thompson S (2005) Is redistribution a form of recognition? Comments on the Fraser-Honneth debate. *Critical Review of International Social and Political Philosophy*, Vol. 8(1): 85-102.

Tracy T J (1969) *Physiological Theory and the Doctrine of the Mean in Plato and Aristotle.* Chicago, IL: Loyola University Press.

Tucker R C (1964) *Philosophy and Myth in Karl Marx.* Cambridge: Cambridge University Press.

Turner B S (2009) *The New Blackwell Companion to Social Theory.* Chichester: Wiley-Blackwell.

Twelve Angry Men. (1957) [Film]. Beverly Hill, CA: MGM.

Tyler L (1990) Bastien und Bastienne: The Libretto, Its Derivation, and Mozart's Text-Setting. *The Journal of Musicology.* 8(4): 520-552.

Van den Brink B (1997) Gesellschaftstheorie und Übertreibungskunst: Für eine Alternative Lesart der 'Dialektik der Aufklärung' ... Die neue Rundschau, 108(1), 37-59.

Vandenberghe F (2013) *What's Critical About Critical Realism? Essays in Reconstructive Social Theory.* Abingdon: Routledge.

Varga S and Gallagher S (2012) Critical Social Theory, Honneth and the role of primary intersubjectivity. *European Journal of Social Theory* 15(2): 243-260.

Viroli M (1988) *Jean-Jacques Rousseau and the 'well-ordered society'.* Translated by Hanson D. Cambridge: Cambridge University Press.

Wells H G (2012 [1904]) *The Country of the Blind.* Stillwell, KS: Digireads.

Whitehead A N (1979) *Process and Reality.* New York City, NY: Free Press.

Wilde L (1998) *Ethical Marxism and its Radical Critics.* London: Palgrave Macmillan.

———. (2004) *Erich Fromm and the Quest for Solidarity.* London: Palgrave Macmillan.

Will H (1984) *Die Geburt der Psychosomatik. Georg Groddeck, der Mensch und Wissenchaftler.* Munich: Urban and Schwarzenberg.

Wilson B (2018) Profiting from Pride. *Exepose.* Available online at: https://exepose.com/2018/07/01/profiting-from-pride/ [Accessed 15th March 2019].

Wilson N (1959) Substances without Substrata. *The Review of Metaphysics.* 12(4) 521-539.

Winnicott D (1965) *The Maturational Process and the Facilitating Environment: Studies in the Theory of Emotional Development.* London: Hogarth Press and the Institute of Pyschoanalysis.

———. (1971) *Playing and Reality.* London: Tavistock.

Wokler R (2001) *Rousseau: A Very Short Introduction.* Oxford: Oxford University Press.

Wood A (1990) *Hegel's Ethical Theory.* New York, NY: Cambridge University Press.

Yack B (1997) *The Fetishism of Modernities: Epochal Self-Consciousness in Contemporary Social and Political Thought.* Notre Dame: University of Notre Dame Press.

Young I M (1990) *Justice and the Politics of Difference.* Princeton, NJ: Princeton University Press.

Younge G (2018) Sajid Javid is change, but don't be fooled. He's not real progress. *The Guardian.* 3rd May 2018. Available online at: https://www.theguardian.com/commentisfree/2018/may/03/sajid-javid-father-immigration-poverty-british-pakistani-tory [Accessed 18th January 2019].

Zurn C (2011) Social Pathologies as second-order disorders. In: Petherbridge D (ed.) *Axel Honneth: Critical Essays: with a reply by Axel Honneth.* Leiden: Brill, pp. 345-370.

CPSIA information can be obtained
at www.ICGtesting.com
Printed in the USA
LVHW080547280223
740519LV00015B/202